I0091231

IS YOUR NEURON BROKE?

Where Counselling Meets Neuroscience

By

ANTHONY ENGEL

The copyright and the rights of translation in any language are reserved by the publishers and copyright owner. No part, passage, text, photograph, or artwork of this book, except for the use of brief quotations in a book review, should be reproduced, transmitted, or utilized, in the original language or by translation, in any form or by any means, electronic, mechanical, photocopying, recording of by any information storage and retrieval system except with the express and prior permission, in writing, from the copyright author.

Copyright © 2020 by Anthony Engel. All rights reserved.

Contact: analyst2@bigpond.com

Editing by Jacob Hansen and Devin Kinser with Hansen Book Consulting (HansenBookConsulting.com) 2020. Edited for audio by Anthony Engel 2023

First Printed October 2015

Reprinted January 2017

Cover Update December 2020

Revised Edition December 2020

ISBN: 978-0-646-83203-6

Author's Note

Please read this book from cover to cover to fully appreciate its contents. Please do not skip to the chapter that interests you because you will miss the entire message of this book. Significant data is dispersed throughout its pages, and you may miss vital information about neuron therapy and the biological science underlying psychotherapy as a consequence.

In addition, numerous people contributed to the creation of this publication. I would like to thank them for their time, shared experiences, and courage. This composition is dedicated to them and everyone else who is willing to investigate new methods for managing their mental health.

Contents

Preface

This book is about neuroscience, which is the study of the nervous system, chiefly the brain and the spinal cord. It entails discovering more about how the mind works. The brain is an amazing organ and can actually change itself to suit its environment and it can make repairs along the way when needed. This is called neuroplasticity.

In this book, you will learn how to tap into the mind and access your inner workings of the brain, in particular, your neurons and neural networks, with the aim of getting hold of these brain cells and making positive changes. You will learn how to unlock your potential and change your mindset to one that is more favourable to your emotional well-being.

Are any of your neurons broken?

Read about real people who share their stories about broken neurons and how these are reflected on the outside. They talk about depression, anxiety, PTSD, addictions and more, and are surprised to learn that by modifying neurons in the brain, changes are made in mood and behaviour as well. By simply rewiring your brain, you can produce the changes you seek.

Disclaimer

This book was written for those people interested in examining new ways to manage their mental health. If you are under the care of a doctor or mental health practitioner and wish to adapt the techniques employed in this book, please discuss with your treating clinician before trying any of the practices in these pages.

This book should not be applied as a backup or surrogate for your mainstream therapy sessions; perhaps used with psychotherapy or when other psychological approaches are not working for you. Still, the contents in this book may not be suitable for your psychiatric needs and should be regarded with caution. As well, this book is not worthy of those people who have trouble distinguishing reality from fantasy, and those who possess limited (or no) capacity for introspection.

Lastly, before reading this book, please practice caution, as the author does not accept any liability for any adverse action or consequence that may arise based on the information provided within this book.

You have to go inside
to free yourself on the outside.

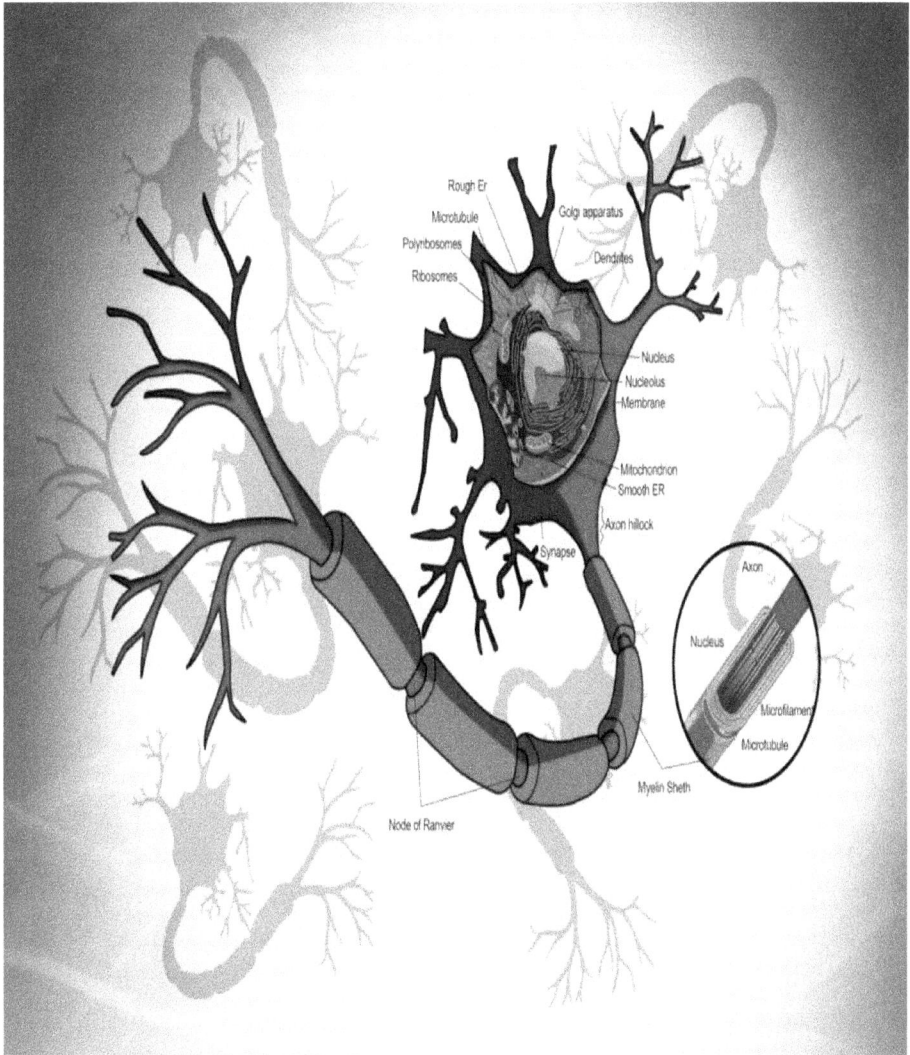

Rough Er
Microtubule
Polyribosomes
Ribosomes
Golgi apparatus
Dendrites
Nucleus
Nucleolus
Membrane
Mitochondrion
Smooth ER
Axon hillock
Synapse
Axon
Nucleus
Microfilament
Microtubule
Myelin Sheth
Node of Ranvier

Letters from Clients

Anxiety

I have been asked to write a brief account of what I think of Neuron Therapy. I am extremely happy to do so, as I have been struggling with anxiety for many years, and at times, I found my condition so unbearable I thought of just disappearing forever!

I have been up and down the mental health road that many in my situation would have also travelled. Meaning, seeing my doctor, and then being referred to psychologists or psychiatrists or both, and after repeating my story over and over, been given medication and on a couple of occasions, they thought I'd be better off hospitalised. I was at the end of my tether. I felt alone and had nothing to look forward to. Was this really my life!? Was I going to be a burden to my family and friends forever? What about a partner? Who on earth would want to be with me, anyway? I am so broken. I really felt alone. It was so scary being me.

Then one day, I'm not sure how this happened, I saw something on TV or perhaps on the internet or maybe I read it somewhere, who knows; when you have a sick mind, you can't recall certain things. From what I do remember, it was about changing your neurons or something about fixing yourself by yourself. Like hacking into your own brain and fixing yourself from the inside. I quickly began researching neuroplasticity and this new science about changing brain chemistry and tapping into the power of the mind. The more I researched, the more excited I became. It's all about mind over matter. One can alter the situation in the brain from a negative or fearful outlook to a more helpful and content mind-set. Sounds so easy but is this true? The Gods must have been on my side that day because I found someone who specializes in this very topic and his rooms were not far from where I lived.

All I can say is that Anthony Engel helped me enormously and I am in his debt forever. I can't believe, and neither can my family, the remarkable change within me. My whole life has turned around and my overactive and fearful mind is no longer present. I can frankly state that I am anxiety free for the first time in as long as I can remember. The very simple tricks and strategies taught to me during my sessions really worked. I still can't get over how simple this was. I also can't understand why this treatment is not made more available to the public.

Neuron Therapy works and I highly recommend this treatment if you are at all experiencing debilitating symptoms of anxiety.

Rhonda – 46 years old

Anxiety with Panic

Hi, Anthony asked me to write the following if I wanted to. I wanted to.

I used to suffer with anxiety and panic. My parents sent me to the doctor because I was getting panicky and sick all the time. The doctor then sent me for further tests, including a colonoscopy. He also thought I may have IBS. I had a brain scan because of my headaches. All my tests came back okay. There was nothing physically wrong with me. The doctor then told my parents that these things may be in my head. Yep, they thought I was crazy. The doctor gave me Zoloft medication and referred me to a shrink.

I ended up seeing Anthony and he fixed me within a short period of time. He was the first psychologist I had ever seen, and I guess I was lucky to see him. We got on well and he taught me heaps. I liked the visualization exercises. Long story short, I do not have anxiety or panic anymore. I do not have IBS anymore. I do not have a nervous bowel anymore. I do not get headaches any longer. And I am no longer on Zoloft.

Cheers

Elliot – 20 years old,

Depression

You've probably heard these stories before. However, this is about me, and I can tell you that I wouldn't be writing this if it wasn't for Anthony. *(I know he doesn't want to hear this. He just wants me to write my own experience with neuron therapy (NT) and not to mention much about him).* However, I am going to mention him, because I have seen many therapists and specialists over the years and I can tell you one thing, a friendly and approachable style is important. Anthony is warm, reassuring, and genuine, and this helped me trust him and travel the sometimes-daunting journey with him. From day one, I learnt about brain neurons and how they work together. And from day one, I knew this wise man was going to help me.

My name is James and I have been struggling with depression and anger and addictions for so many years. I drink alcohol and smoke cigarettes to cope with my depressed moods. I have seen endless counsellors and doctors over the years and have been prescribed all sorts of antidepressants, and yet there has been minimal or no improvement.

My partner at the time dragged me to see Anthony as I was reluctant to venture near any more so-called professionals. I am no longer with my partner, but to this day I want to thank her for having the motivation to get me into therapy.

When I met Anthony, as mentioned previously, I noticed a remarkable difference in how he works. He zeroed in on my moods very quickly and within a short time, he knew how my mind worked. When he talked about NT, I was happy to try anything. I had already lost partners, friends, and my job was hanging by a thread.

Neuron Therapy, which I understand is explained in this book, really works. It just shows you how powerful your mind can be. The greatest shock to me was discovering that I could change or adjust the way my brain works. I could alter the wiring and firing of my own brain cells. Additionally, I could influence serotonin, oxytocin and dopamine levels in my brain and visualize any outcome I wished to accomplish. All along I had this power within me. As Anthony says, it's all about mind over matter, and it really works!

My depression has lifted. My anger is gone. My mood, fantastic. I have a new girlfriend and she finds it hard to believe that I suffered with depression. My life is back, and I am happy.

James – 37 years old.

Introduction

This book is an uncomplicated and easy-to-read guide on neuroplasticity and how this new science is revolutionizing mental health around the globe. Put simply, this book is about the neurons in your brain and how these cells influence your daily life. Nerve cells (neurons) that fire together, wire happily together. Neurons that fire apart, sadly wire apart, also causing stress and other problems for the unsuspecting individual. This is where neuroscience plays a great part in realizing how your brain communicates on a cellular level. Normal firing neurons will bring about content people and broken neurons will contribute to faulty thinking patterns and behaviours that may be debilitating for the individual. On these pages, however, I will be focusing primarily on mental health issues and how neuroplasticity can help in addressing these sometimes-incapacitating conditions.

In this book, you will find out how to modify and change existing brain neurons to manage your mental health. You will find out how to rid yourself of those faulty and unhelpful thinking patterns that are constantly holding you back and stopping you from reaching your full potential as a social, contributing and satisfied human being.

Find out how these neurons work and how they can influence your life from a psychological and emotional perspective. Many think that this neuroplasticity approach is the 'missing link' when it comes to psychology. Altering and modifying your brain neurons can bring about positive changes in your mental health that you never imagined possible.

Neuroscience is essentially the subject area of the neural system, however, in this book, I will be focusing on neuroplasticity; zeroing in on brain cells, in particular, that play a major role in our emotions. Neuroplasticity is about the brain's ability to reorganize itself by forging new neural networks and connectors on a continuing basis, making modifications where necessary to conform to changes in the surroundings. Also, when needed, brain neurons can grow new nerve endings to connect to other neurons. You can usually see this with injury or disease. Our mind is wired to be pliable and malleable or plastic, meaning that we can fix and alter neurons with our free will and intellect. It just requires some 'mental' elbow grease on our behalf.

The term Neuroplasticity comes from the words Neuron and Plastic. A neuron (focusing on brain neurons) refers to the nerve cells in the brain. Each of these neural cells is constructed of an axon and a dendrite and is connected by a little space called a synapse. See Diagram on page 57. The word plastic means to alter, transform, change and so on. That means that neuroplasticity refers to the possibility that the brain can modify itself by reorganizing new neural networks when needed. Many researchers in neuroscience believe that the brain has the power to change or mold itself to fit varying situations or for the chief intent of matching the individual's needs, whatever that may be for him or her, good or bad or for love or evil.

This is where neuroscience becomes exciting. The research out there proposes that you can change your neurons and neural networks through counselling, visualization, and other sorts of guided therapy. So, if you believe you can, you can. You are what you think, or what you have programmed yourself to be.

Is it possible to regrow, say damaged neural networks? Is it possible to fix and repair damaged neurons from years of faulty and negative thinking patterns or from something more horrific, such as a traumatic experience? Actually, can damaged neurons be fixed? What about the genetic debate about inheriting impaired or faulty genes from our parents and ancestors? Is it possible to mend or rebuild those defective neurons handed down unintentionally to us? Well, studies out there tell us we can! From a psychiatric approach, this is awesome news. Neuroplasticity and Psychotherapy have come out of the research laboratories and are now being used around the world by competent psychologists and other mental health clinicians. Many of these treating mental health experts are reporting outstanding results for their patients. I have also noticed significant changes in my own clients when I incorporated this approach into their treatment programs.

In this manuscript, I will be presenting a few significant instances, real-life people that have given permission for me to narrate their stories. You will learn for yourself how neuroplasticity works and how this approach, along with other treatments, worked together to bring about monumental changes in many of my clients' lives. Even the most challenging and long-term cases produced positive results when neuron therapy was introduced.

I also want to mention that I felt humbled during the process of putting this book together, as many of my past and existing clients wanted to be part of this book and have their tales told. Many of my clients had endured several years of therapy with various clinicians and, once they were finally introduced to neuroplasticity and neuron therapy, and had these approaches incorporated into their therapy sessions, significant and rapid changes took place.

Many of my former clients continue to live rich and contented lives, experiencing a whole new understanding and awareness of how their minds work. Many have learned how to handle their lives from a quantum perspective, by modifying and changing brain neurons from within, to form healthy neural networks, thus creating significant changes on the outside.

I have been studying and researching neuroplasticity for many years now, however, I only introduced this therapeutic approach to my clients about four and a half years ago, since the date of writing this book. I wanted to be certain that this new science was legitimate and had been supported by many experts in the neuroscience area. I have been cognizant of this exceptional field of psychology for many years – over twenty, possibly more, and have always been intrigued by the brain and its many layers and functions of brain cells to complex neural nets. Frustratingly though, we are just scraping the surface of understanding the human mind. Nevertheless, thanks to neuroscience, we now understand the emotional and biological brain in more detail than ever before.

As cited previously, when I first introduced this approach to my clientele group, I decided to hand-pick individual cases, those who I assessed as being able to accept this new and revolutionary approach to overseeing their respective mental health worries. I have also realized that there are a few people that do not react well to neuroplasticity through psychotherapy, as they had trouble grasping the visualization and sometimes repetitious techniques needed to influence rewiring on the cellular stage. They had trouble with going inside to produce results on the outside. Thus, sadly, not everyone will benefit from this new and creative approach.

I trust that you will find this area of science fascinating as I believe neuroplasticity will not just revolutionize how we treat psychological disorders in the future but will eventually become the 'norm' when treating people's mental health concerns.

Anthony Engel

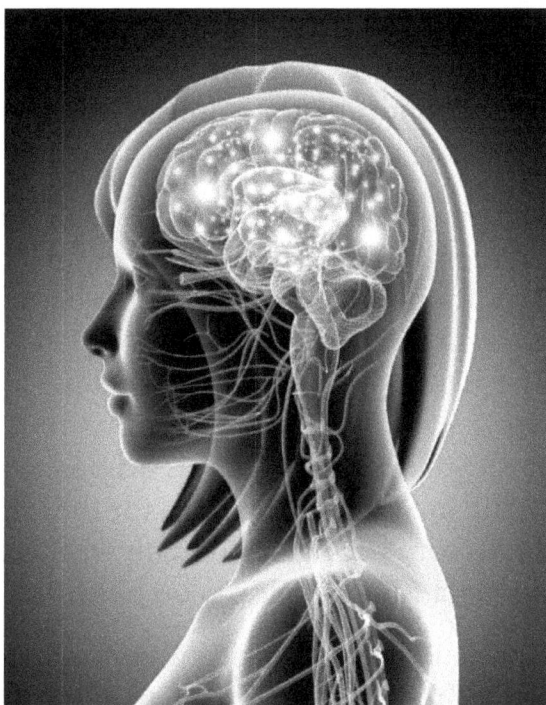

CHAPTER ONE:
When East Meets West

Cynthia's Story (Age mid-forties)

Cynthia was angry on the inside.

First off, what is the meaning of culture? Most of us are aware of the many differences between civilizations from one country to another—social and religious habits and so on. What about genetics or workplace culture? Is culture characterized by a group of people defined by their differences, such as language, customs, values, and habits? There is no one answer to these questions. We human beings are similarly complicated and too ever-changing to come up with the single correct solution that will satisfy everyone reading this book. Even so, read along and find out for yourself the result of Cynthia's anxiety-producing story.

In this chapter, we will focus on Cynthia's belief system and personal values, as these are the result of her cultural upbringing. I often remember her words because they still ring in my head today. When I first met Cynthia, she said: "It's the injustice that gets me. How can they treat me like this?" She was referring to her work situation. Cynthia (not her real name) lived not far from my office but was originally from China. She has been living in Sydney, Australia, for the last nineteen years. She separated from her husband many years earlier and raised her two Australian-born children on her own.

Cynthia claimed that she had always experienced what she referred to as "mild anxiety," but that she had to make do because she was a working professional and a single mother. Her anxiety had, however, been increasing lately. She confided in me that she was finding it difficult to adjust to the radical and rapid changes at work. She added that she thought her new manager was a bully and that the recent, significant changes the business had made had left her with a negative impression of her manager and the company she was working for. Cynthia said they went against her personal convictions and ran counter to her fundamental values and moral principles. She had a lot of trouble implementing the changes they wanted her to make. Cynthia even thought of harming herself especially when she felt totally overwhelmed and exhausted by her unpredictable and ever-increasing workload.

Although we can sympathize with Cynthia, I want to focus on how her upbringing and cultural background are impacting both her current situation at work and her personal life as well. When we reached the skills training section of her treatment plan, I noticed the cultural influences coming into play.

Cynthia struggled with being assertive and less passive. In other words, with speaking up and voicing her concerns to management. But according to Cynthia, her Asian background did not approve of speaking up and negotiating with one's superiors. She believed in a hierarchical order and knew her place as a subordinate in relation to the managers above her. So, assertiveness training went out the door. Passivity remained Cynthia's default position, for now. And as usual, Cynthia swallowed up her anger and kept it neatly packed away, deep within her being, all the while soldiering on as normal. Now and again, resentment poured forth, but she continued with her daily commitments as a dutiful employee and mother. At times, she did feel those dark moments when she believed she would be better off dead but reassured me that she would never leave her daughters in that way.

This is merely one of the many cases showing how cultural issues can negatively affect the healing process when the worldview of the counsellor is different from that of the client. The therapist needs to be skilled in this area for there to be a good result for the client. Finding the middle ground, or a solution to move forward, is paramount. As you read along, you will see for yourself how we accomplished this.

Let us move on to the inherited stuff for a moment. These are genes handed down to us by our parents. The *BBS*! Meaning, the Big Biological Stuff! These genes can be healthy or not so healthy. The not-so-healthy genes may be defective or carry with them disease or other problems that may bring about behavioural and or physical problems for the individual. Or, put another way, there appears to be more challenges for these people to overcome in terms of managing their psychological (and physical) deficiencies.

Were Cynthia's neurons firing properly? Was she handed down any genes that needed more scrutiny? Remember, she did mention that she had always experienced modest anxiety, but she blamed her current workplace for her anxiety peaking. Let's go inside her head for a moment.

Because of the ongoing external trauma going on in her workplace—working long hours, feeling uncertain of her role, being bullied, not speaking up and voicing her concerns, and so on—were these situations all being acted out in her brain on a cellular level as well? Were her neurons and neural networks reacting to those outside influences and conflicting messages in a negative fashion, thus causing them to become energetic? Sometimes these neurons and brain cells may take on a survival role, envisioning danger on the outside and going into survival mode on the inside. If they go into survival mode, an increase of energy will occur and the firing of neurons will also increase, causing a sense of urgency and super awareness, pushing, or compelling the body to keep up with the speeding brain. Imagine this: A person is running as fast as they can, trying to catch their speeding brain that is racing outside their head, about two or three feet in front of their body. This is what happens when people are feeling overwhelmed, anxious, and reactive. Their brain waves and millions of neurons become elevated.

Were the problems in the workplace also affecting her neurons on a cellular level as well? Were her brain cells and neural networks responding negatively to those outside stimuli and conflicting messages, making them more agitated? When there is danger outside, these neurons and brain cells will become alert and trigger the release of stress hormones. If a person enters internal survival mode, their energy levels will increase as their bodies are placed on high alert, generating a sense of urgency and heightened awareness. When a person feels threatened or sense danger, they experience this condition. In an effort to protect the physical body, the amygdala, a portion of the brain, reacts instantaneously to threats. It does so in two ways: by fighting or by acting lifeless.

This natural process will occur when the individual is in danger, as the body goes into action to save itself. In Cynthia's case, the opposite occurs. There is no outside *(or real)* danger, only what is transpiring in her head. Cynthia's anticipatory thinking *(the constant fear of what is going to happen next in her unpredictable workplace),* is activating her survival systems. Moreover, extreme thinking patterns, considered negative and faulty, will also trigger the chemical chain reaction of turning on Cynthia's fight and flight response system which, in turn, will cause her to experience a peak in her anxiety, thus causing her body to lose vital energy *(as the body gears up for survival purposes, it will take energy from other parts of the body).* That energy will now be prioritized to be used to stabilize Cynthia's over-active mind and sympathetic nervous system. And throughout, there is no external threat, only disquieting chemical messages emanating from Cynthia's own fearful thought patterns regarding what might occur next in her stressful workplace.

Simply put, Cynthia's stress and anxiety levels were significantly affected by the fact that she was not speaking out in her workplace, accepting all the injustice and unfairness, keeping quiet, and pretending that she was pleased with her work situation when clearly, she was not. Her constant, excessive worry about her predicament led to a hyper-anxious mindset and mood swings, which affected her capacity to control her emotions. Her fight-or-flee response systems were constantly engaged as she was in a condition of survival. Cynthia was in a constant state of struggle with herself, and her body was now acting in a way to reflect this.

Cynthia had compromised her morals, her outlook, and her laid-back personality because of all this. She was losing hope, happiness, and herself; she was filled with repressed rage and resentment. She was no longer in charge of her life. She was a victim being pulled along in someone else's chaotic world; she was no longer the creator or the one in control of her existence. Her body (brain and sympathetic nervous system) was interpreting these cues as danger signals and deciding to enter survival mode to defend itself. And keep in mind, our brains are not able to tell the difference between what is occurring outside and what one is imagining (or interpreting) on the inside. Whether a dangerous animal is ready to attack you, or you are simply sitting there fantasizing that you are about to be mauled by a ferocious beast, the same hormonal reactions will take place regardless of whether the threat is real or just imagined; the same brain circuitry will activate. In Cynthia's case, anxiety and stress made themselves known by manifesting physical symptoms because of her worrisome situation in her workplace. Remember, what you think, or interpret, will become a reality in your mind and your emotional and biological body will respond accordingly.

Cynthia stated that she was not aware of any faulty genes being passed down to her and questioned whether her current state of distress was a result of something new, either environmental or brought on by stress at work. In either case, sustained stress will have a deleterious effect on her brain cells and may cause her to respond by withdrawing or shutting down. As previously mentioned, if her brain's neurons are functioning normally, they should be sending and receiving messages via chemical and electrical impulses from neuron to neuron, across the synapse junction to the next neuron, and so on. The outside world will also be in good shape if these neurons are firing cheerfully and efficiently. However, a low mood is typically reported if these nerve cells are not firing properly, are broken, or are somehow disrupted. But, if on the other hand, these neurons are overactive, firing and wiring too quickly, as they were in Cynthia's instance, anxiety can be present. The physical and observable world reflects what occurs here at the cellular level. Depending on the state of the person's inner world of neurons, these expressions may turn out to be either negative or positive for them.

I'll return to Cynthia's case later. You can see for yourself as you read on how this woman changed her inner reality via the application of neuroplasticity and psychotherapy, thereby realizing her full potential in the outside world.

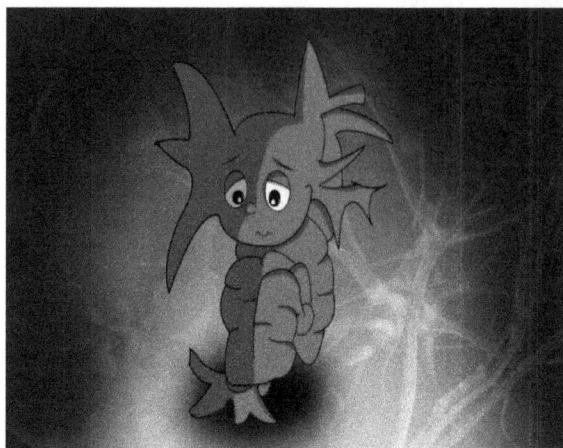

CHAPTER TWO:
When Daydreaming Becomes Your Best Friend

Ben's Story (Age 9)

This is a story of Attention Deficit Disorder

Ben was becoming increasingly distant.

Attention Deficit Disorder (ADD) or Attention Deficit Hyperactivity Disorder (ADHD) is another one of those areas the neuroscientists are getting excited about. Is ADD genetic, environmental, or perhaps a combination of the two? Or is it something else altogether?

Ben was a nine-year-old who was presented alongside his concerned and worried parents. They were convinced that he had ADD. The doctor had told them so. The teacher had her suspicions and referrals were made. The pediatrician confirmed it. A private psychologist was recruited and she also, in a roundabout way, confirmed that young Ben may indeed be suffering with ADD, but was reluctant to write the diagnosis down. Not ADHD but ADD. (Seemingly, there was no hyperactivity when it came to Ben. But it seems that nowadays many clinicians do not draw a distinction between the two terms anymore, only stating hyperactivity, if present, with an ADD diagnosis.)

The three primary characteristics of ADD and ADHD are inattention, hyperactivity, and impulsivity.

Young Ben, nine years old, turned up with his excessively eager mother and a concerned, but silent father. They reported that Ben was having difficulties concentrating and maintaining attention, that he was not listening to their instructions or following simple directions. He was easily distracted, often avoided or was reluctant to engage in any activities needing mental effort, and frequently lost his belongings, which were of great concern to his parents because some of these items were expensive. Because of Ben's frustrations and, realizing that something may be amiss with him, he set about acting out and became aggressive and wild.

Regarding his schoolwork, Ben had become withdrawn and anxious about his poor academic performance, as other youngsters were now teasing him and calling him terrible names due to his failings. He began realizing that it was not normal to keep losing expensive items, and not only that, but the other children in his grade were brighter, more in command of their emotions, and often got high marks in their exams, where he frequently failed. Ben became distant and started isolating himself from his peers.

It took a few sessions for Ben's parents to update me with their thoughts about their son before I started working with young Ben alone. It took a few more sessions before a rapport developed between us. Ben was shy at first, but slowly warmed into the sessions and got used to the process, coming with his father after school on a weekly, then fortnightly basis. I also educated his parents on parenting skills for managing their son's behaviour.

With the help of art therapy, a modified version of cognitive behaviour therapy, and skills training with a focus on assertiveness and resilience-building, a treatment plan tailored to the patient's age was put into place. Relaxation techniques were also taught. In an effort to explain to Ben why he behaved the way he did and the causes of his moods and actions, we drew diagrams together indicating helpful thinking versus unhelpful thinking. He was very self-conscious, so trying roleplaying did not go well at first. However, after turning the role play into an unscripted comedic show, a young celebrity eventually emerged.

I'm happy to report that Ben has improved and was better aware of his thought process. He now had a better understanding of his *scary thinking side* (ST) and his *rational thinking side* (RT), and he was aware that he could choose between the two. The big RT versus the big ST. To reinforce his new thought patterns, we used these names by their initials. Additionally, it concealed the phrase's true meaning—that young boys are all about playing games and keeping harmless secrets. He did not want others to know the real meaning behind these words. When we used the initials, Ben immediately understood how he was thinking.

Ben also realized that he was excessively daydreaming and squandering valuable 'doing time,' and he began to become more action oriented. He could now choose independently which mode of thought to employ in each circumstance. He now had the ability and resources to choose between his old way of thinking and his new and improved way of thinking. His parents had observed substantial changes in their son, and they were, to say the least, impressed, and ecstatic. Counselling was effective! And Ben's overly anxious parents could now move on from this difficult period of their lives. Or could they? We will return to young Ben a bit later in this book, and you will see for yourself what happened next. The tale does not end here...

The Mind is everything.
What you think you become.

Buddha

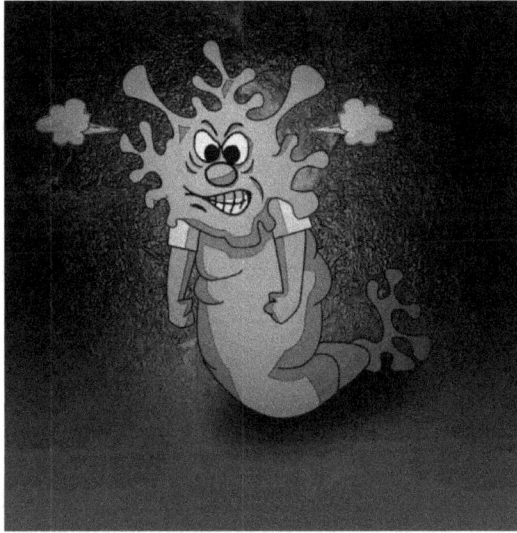

CHAPTER THREE:
Sixteen Going on to Two

Stephen's Story (Age 16)

This is a story of Anxiety and Anger

Stephen locked horns with everyone.

Let's call this young man, Stephen. He and his mother presented for counselling one hot afternoon after his school had ended. It was February and summer in Sydney. I remembered how hot it was that day and Stephen arrived in an irritable mood. They came into my counselling room and his mother did most of the talking, as Stephen sat on, watching his mother and me, with a disapproving look on his face. It was obvious, Stephen did not wish to be in the session and gave the feeling that he was uncomfortable, as he listened to what his mother was saying about him. She happily hung out the dirty laundry about her son's conduct, not holding anything back. At one moment, an argument broke out between them. I heard Stephen say in a grumpy voice that his mother was exaggerating and telling lies about his behaviour.

Eventually, Stephen's mother reported symptoms consistent with a generalized anxiety disorder (GAD) with panic symptoms. She also reported that he was an angry young man, but she was unaware of the source of his wrath. In the past, he was a cheerful, entertaining, and loving child, but recently he had become a vile monster.

The second time Stephen saw me by himself, he was upset. His mother had threatened to send him to her strict older brother who lived on a farm in the country if he did not go to counselling. There were just lush green woodlands and cows in that region, so it was obvious that there was no Internet or mobile phone coverage. Stephen swiftly scheduled a meeting with me. The tension between them increased when his mother contacted my office to inquire if he had arrived.

Many may be wondering if there is more to these stories than meets the eye. In other words, could there be other disorders other than the cultural differences as in Chapter One, or ADD in Chapter Two or anxiety as mentioned earlier? Some may reflect that anger management may be an issue; what about depression and even a conduct disorder—perhaps the early onset of psychosis? I agree. I do work holistically, and I am aware of the many co-occurring disorders that may be present. However, you will examine how all these symptoms are tied together and are not just linked to one disorder but sometimes, many.

Stephen's mother, Elizabeth, often used this phrase: 'Sixteen going on to two', to describe his behaviour at times. Two is the age some parents often cite as the 'terrible twos' in two-year-old youngsters, as they test their limits. Stephen's mother told me on four separate occasions that Stephen resorted to acting like a youngster when he could not get his way. Stephen is clearly not a happy camper. He disliked everyone: his mother, school, teachers, some acquaintances and even himself. Occasionally, I got it too!

In his later sessions with me, Stephen was remarkably talkative and not moody or angry, which was surprising. At the time of his first consultation with me, he was wretched. The third time he met with me, his demeanour altered, and he was courteous. This was a significant shift. I wondered if he was playing games, hoping that if he presents well, I may just tell him that he doesn't have to see me again. But I would eventually find out that he was keen to attend therapy because, after his sessions with me, he would then wander about in town, catching up with friends, and seeing the places adolescents visit when in the big city. He would then go home later than usual, and his mother could not say anything. After all, he was seeing the counsellor in town, and the buses were late again.

Over time, Stephen developed a greater interest in therapy, particularly the psycho-educational portion of the session. He was interested in learning more about his brain's functioning and the reasons for his actions. He admitted to me that he had not anticipated counselling to be that enlightening and fantastic. He also exhibited curiosity in how the sexes differ in terms of psychology and thought processes. He had observed the female students in his class at school and discovered that they were more talkative than the boys and had a greater grasp of social issues.

Unfortunately, Stephen did not take to cognitive behavioural therapy (CBT) too easily, and I had to try to present it in a more creative fashion for his understanding and interest. Briefly, CBT is a type of psychotherapy that helps people to change negative or unhealthy thinking habits, feelings, and behaviours. But Stephen preferred skills training instead, along with role plays, keeping journals and weekly planners, so he could be accountable for what he had achieved for that week. He liked the practical stuff—wanting to see the result and reward in real-time, not interested in psycho-jumbo talk, as he puts it. The big PJ talk! The reward system worked well for Stephen, and he also thrived when it came to the personal development side of things, focusing on identity and personal values, which he was only now discovering about himself.

Nearly six months had passed, and you couldn't get Stephen away from counselling. He even talked about becoming a psychologist himself. He was intrigued by the science and psychology of the human mind. There was also a remarkable improvement in his mood. Gone was the resentful and angry young man that tormented his mother whenever he felt frustrated about himself, and gone was the unhappy, anxious, and panicky adolescent that didn't care about anyone or anything. His mother had finally got her son back, and they were happy. But things change. They say adolescence is a tumultuous stage to go through, but what happened next with Stephen will not only astonish you but shock you. From one neuron to another, as you will eventually see, something from out of the blue swooped down and threw a giant spanner into Stephen's works. Sometimes, just when you believe you've reached the end of a dark and lonely tunnel, you see a light in the distance, only to discover to your horror that it's not the exit to freedom, but a high-speed train speeding towards you.

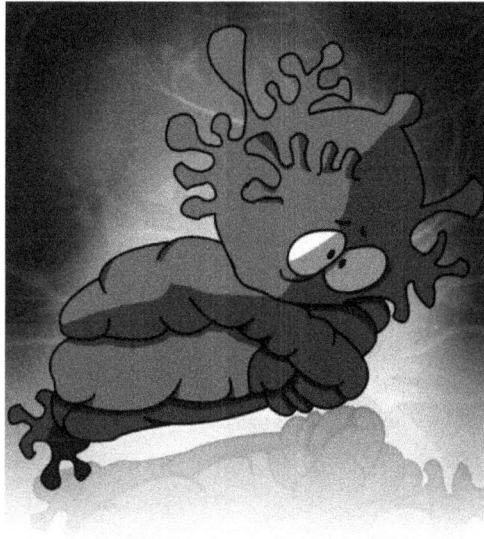

CHAPTER FOUR:
The Black Dog Wouldn't Let Me Go

Patrick's Story (Age mid-thirties)

This is a story about Depression

Patrick had just about given up on life...

Patrick is a man, in his mid-thirties and married. They have a two-year-old little boy. They live in the outer suburbs of town and are both hardworking people. They are financially secure and doing the best they can at living and getting on with life. But Patrick harbours a dark secret. Depression. These were his words when he first came to see me. Hardly anybody knows about his depression because he keeps it under wraps. His wife knows of his low moods and miserable attitude, which was putting pressure on their relationship. Patrick feared he may be judged or may not make that job promotion if his managers found out about his melancholia. He has seen his doctor over the years and was prescribed medication. He tells me his medication is a low dosage and he manages his moods by eating healthy, sleeping regular hours, and exercising. When he feels down, he avoids people altogether so no one will see him in his depressed state. He reported that he feels listless, unmotivated, confused, mind going blank, or lingering on negative thoughts of doom and gloom. He becomes teary for no obvious reason and sometimes feels as if he is better off away from his family and from everyone and everything. He told me with tears rolling down his face that he had lost interest in everything that matters, including life itself.

Patrick is a deeply private man, and the idea of counselling was not in his makeup. Mental health problems were not in his mind-set either, and so he referred to his depression as a dark secret and a sign of weakness. According to him, counselling was for fragile and overly sensitive people, particularly for adult females and possibly children. Not for men! He said that if he couldn't help himself, no one else could. He also believed that men should keep their feelings to themselves, full stop! Talking about his feelings would not make any difference and would only make him feel worse, he told me. He believed in the 'out of mind, out of sight' expression. In other words, if you don't blab about it, it will disappear.

I recollect, we were a few weeks into therapy, when I had discovered some positive changes in Patrick, however, a few weeks afterward, he was down again, and he felt defeated and tired. He told me on many occasions that I was flogging a dead horse and couldn't understand why I had faith in him; why I was so optimistic that he would eventually learn how to manage his depression and be content with life again? After all, he had already given up on happiness over a year ago. This pattern repeated itself over the months, with Patrick feeling in control and a little motivated for a time, but then falling back into days of deep depression. His prognosis was not looking too good. But unknown to Patrick, just around the corner, something wonderful was about to happen to him. He was about to find a fresh way of thinking and managing his depression. For the first time, he was beginning to agree with me that I was no longer flogging a dead horse, but a horse desperate to get up and do some flogging of its own. For the first time in a long while, I was seeing hope in his sad blue eyes, and enthusiasm trying to form an entrance, albeit awkwardly and nervously, through his bodily mannerisms. Even so, optimism had finally arrived. Patrick was standing tall, quick to conquer anyone and anything. So, may we ask the question? What on earth did Patrick discover? When you study his story, the hairs at the back of your neck will stand on end when you realize exactly how powerful the mind can be. With some coaching, his brain neurons were prompted to change their 'faulty' messages, to bring about a new way of thinking, which eventually rescued Patrick from the misery of that tortuous black dog.

Who looks outside, dreams;
who looks inside, awakes.

Carl Jung

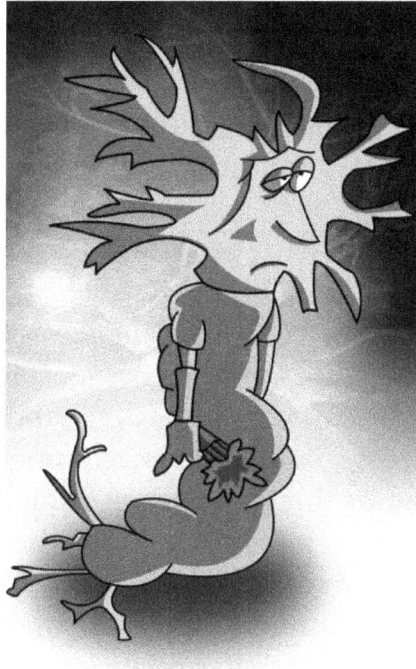

CHAPTER FIVE:
Always the Bridesmaid but Never the Bride

Jacquie's Story (Age thirties)

This is a story about Stress and Mood Swings

Jacquie tends to be impulsive...

Meet Jacquie, a vibrant and vivacious thirty-something year old professional. Jacquie (not her real name) is a busy, skilled, and intelligent person, who lives in an expensive apartment and travels often for her job. Jacquie is a capable, strong-minded, and a beautiful woman who is on the crown of her game. She has many female acquaintances; many of which are lifelong friends. Jacquie should have been happy, but she was profoundly upset about something, and she had become resentful. She also found that she was becoming teary and not wanting to catch up with her friends anymore. Many of them had married and started their families. Jacquie was beginning to think that her friends and colleagues were talking behind her back about why she was still single. They knew she was a heterosexual woman who had dated handsome and successful men over the years, but to no benefit; nothing long-term came from those relationships. Her relationships always broke down. Jacquie could now predict the result when dating a new man. Talk about creating a self-fulfilling prophecy. She would give them a couple of months, depending on how often she would see them, and then watch her relationship end. She reported to me on one occasion, that it was like seeing a car crash in slow-motion. And she was the car!

What was Jacquie doing so wrong? Why couldn't she find a man—and keep him?

I will continue with her story later, and you will be surprised at what this intelligent and caring woman was doing so wrong when it came to finding that man and marrying him.

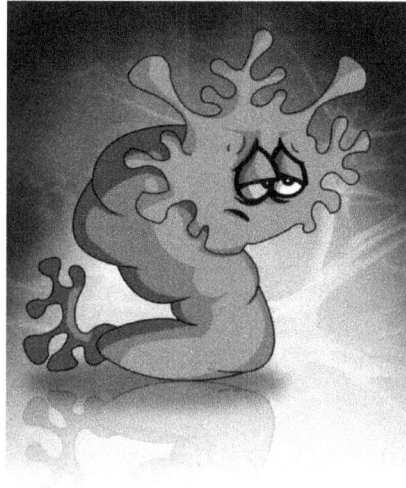

CHAPTER SIX:
Stuck in the Moment of Horror!

Matthew's Story (Age thirties)

This is a story of Anxiety with Post Traumatic Stress Disorder (PTSD)

Matthew was convinced that he was cursed.

Matthew presented in my rooms looking like he had given up on life and was desperate for answers to his mental condition. He looked ragged and worn out, defeated and on the edge of lunacy. He told me he didn't know why he even made the appointment because no one has helped him in the past.

Matthew had not always been like this. He described a happy-go-lucky guy who had become a pathetic shadow of his joyful past. He had given up on relationships, his career, and was now trying to survive financially, while managing his torturous mind. Matthew had been diagnosed with anxiety with posttraumatic stress disorder (PTSD), and lately, his insomnia had gotten worse, along with signs of depression. Sometimes depression develops as a symptom of anxiety or conversely if one is left untreated.

Originally, Matthew was a happy young man and popular in high school. He was well on his way to becoming a solicitor, an occupation he had idolized since his early teens. During a school outing when he was in year ten, aged around sixteen, he participated in boat races down some fast-paced rapids, competing with fellow students as part of the activities for the day. One moment he was laughing with his friends, then without warning, their boat tumbled over after colliding with a submerged rock, toppling Matthew, and his fellow pupils into the raging, icy cold, torrents. They were swept, bouncing up and down in the swell, down the river, many of them grabbed onto debris, rocks, and other rubble along the edges before pulling themselves onto land. This was a disturbing moment for young Matthew, as he just about made it to the water's edge, exhausted, before dragging his tired and shivering body onto solid ground. He was shedding blood, as he'd received many cuts from being dashed against the sharp rocks. His closest friend tragically drowned that day. He did not make it out of the water, and his face-down corpse was discovered floating further down the river. Matthew did not know how to feel or what to do and completely shut down. He went into shock. He did not attend school for nearly a month after that incident and his mood worsened rapidly. He was hospitalized and prescribed medication. In the months that followed, he was treated by psychiatrists and other mental health professionals. That day, he told me, something clicked in his mind, while updating me on his story. He claimed he had never been the same since that day. Still, life continues. He persevered, forging his way in life, graduating from high school, and enrolling in college.

Eventually, Matthew had to find a job to supplement his income while he was in university. He was able to secure a part-time position serving customers in the evenings at a liquor store. Then, one night, just before closing time, he and a female employee were attacked by four armed robbers wearing black balaclavas and carrying long-bladed knives and a pistol as they ran into the vacant store. They cornered the two frightened employees and pointed the gun at Matthew's head while yelling for him to unlock the safe. His colleague fought with one of the robbers before being violently tossed to the concrete floor. Matthew feared the worst when she remained immobile after that.

Over the following months, Matthew became overcautious and stayed away from anything he sensed as dangerous or life-endangering. He told me that he must be cursed or had done something bad in a former life, as he couldn't get over the so-called bad luck he had worn since high school. "Why me?" He often remarked. He had found that alcohol and marijuana worked well to ease his overactive, hyper-vigilant and scary-thinking brain. He discovered that he was no longer able to concentrate well and did not want to be burdened with stressful activities such as continuing to study, participating in hobbies, making the effort to meet new people, or going out with friends. Everything became an annoyance for him, and he desired solitude. Consequently, he quit his part-time employment. He then ensured that no one would bother him by isolating himself in his small apartment.

Matthew continued to relive the horror of that night over and over in his mind. He also found that he was not only reliving the horror of the robbery, but now the death of his best friend all those years ago when he was sixteen. Matthew told me that it was like he was stuck in the moment of those horrors. His co-worker at the liquor store did not die. She made a full 'physical' recovery after treatment.

Meanwhile, he added, he had to work as he had no money. His savings had dwindled over the years. He did basic jobs in secure places, such as office work and answering telephone calls. His pursuit of becoming a solicitor had left him that night when he was robbed and assaulted. He now worked from home most days on his computer, doing basic administrative work for companies. He drank alcohol and smoked cannabis nearly every day, justifying his dependency because it allowed him to sleep at night. He did this for many years until his physical health began to decline. He also noted that he was spending way too much money on his vices, falling way behind with his now limited finances. Lonely, broken, and slowly becoming insane, he finally reached out to his doctor.

Matthew was suffering with PTSD and had acquired an addiction along the way because of his anxious mind-set and horrific past experiences. He tried counselling when he was in his late teens and again temporarily in his twenties when he was robbed and attacked at the liquor store. Now, in his thirties, he decided to try counselling again, on doctor's advice, as he had reached the end of his troubled and lonely road. Matthew had hit rock bottom.

Was it too late for this troubled individual? He was constantly intoxicated and/or high and lacked motivation to improve his situation. However, as you continue reading about this man under siege, you will be inspired to move mountains yourself. What occurred next might remain in your memory forever?

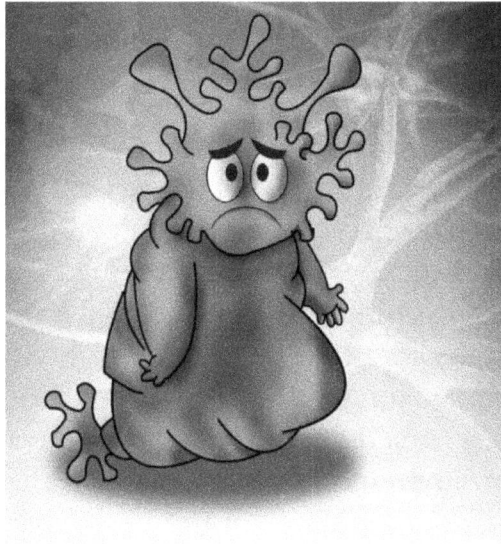

CHAPTER SEVEN:
Eating Towards Happiness

Cassandra's Story (Age twenties)

This is a story about obesity

Cassandra tended to comfort eat more than usual.

Cassandra is a yo-yo when it comes to weight and dress sizes. This is what she told me. One moment Cassandra was satisfied with her weight and the next moment she was ready to scream as the weight reappeared, as if by magic. I remembered Cassandra telling me when we first met, that even if she drank a little glass of water, she would lay on one kilogram of weight. Obviously, this is an overstatement, but this was the frustration this woman has carried every day of her life since her early teen years. She is twenty-three years old and studying part-time at university. She doesn't know what she wants to study and is yet to make up her mind about her career path. She works in a pie shop part-time to complement her earnings.

Cassandra's parents had separated when she was six years old. She has a younger brother, two years younger. The divorce was not a pleasant experience for young Cassandra, and she recalled them arguing constantly. Her parents lived separately and as she got older, she remembered how they argued over the telephone, over payments for her and her brother. Her mother often cursed her father, and vice versa. She loved her father and mother and felt torn by whom she should like more and spend time with. She continued to live with her mother and younger brother and visited her father on the other side of town every two weeks or so.

Also, Cassandra struggled with managing her weight, and because of her faulty thinking patterns, as well as her habits, she would eat junk food frequently, and then try to starve herself later. She also examined all the known diets on the market and spent a lot of money on exercise classes and the gymnasium. But as always, she would be committed at first and then after a week or three, find herself comfort eating in her bedroom late at night. She also enjoyed takeaway food and often overdid that with the promise of never eating junk food again as she binged, justifying to herself that this would be the final time she ate such unhealthy foods. She would say to herself, 'Tomorrow my diet will start.'

Cassandra often gave the impression that she did not know what she wanted and was confused about her identity and where she was heading in life. She has a small group of friends and told me that she is worried about them going their separate ways as they are not as close as they once were when at school. 'Everyone is changing and moving on.' She stated. Cassandra didn't show much interest in boys and when she did, it was short-lived, and she did not want to talk about it. Cassandra seems to be doing everything on her own, such as going to the movies, shopping and even going away on holidays. On her return from one such holiday, Cassandra didn't have much to say about her trip away, only showing me photos, she took on her phone of the wildlife and the ocean. She was becoming a loner, beginning to eat in secret, then starving herself to lose the excess weight.

As you continue reading, it will become apparent that Cassandra used comfort eating to bury unresolved issues from her past and to cope with her increasing stress around her weight gain. You will later learn what transpired and how neuron therapy helped this woman.

*Nothing changes if
nothing changes.*

CHAPTER EIGHT:
Neuroscience

Neuroplasticity

This is a summary of Neuroscience and Neuroplasticity

Neuroscience

Neuroscience is the study of the nervous system, chiefly the brain and the spinal cord. It entails discovering more about how the mind works through the scientific study of the nervous system, and the understanding of how evolving properties of neurons and neural circuits communicate. There are many disciplines associated with neuroscience, such as molecular biology, mathematical modelling, physiology, anatomy, psychology and so on. Quantum Biology is yet another area that plays a role in the understanding of biological processes, especially in the conversion of energy into usable chemical messages, on a quantum level or from a quantum mechanical perspective. Moreover, some quantum scientists speculate that quantum mechanics play a significant role in the living cell, but to what degree, they still don't know. Research in this arena is starting to recognize that the quantum world plays a far bigger part in our nerve cells and their connections than we ever imagined was possible. I also believe that current research in this area will ultimately demonstrate the science behind neuron therapy.

The brain is an amazing organ and holds properties that we have yet to see. It has many layers of awareness, consciousness, unconsciousness and more, which we are just now starting to understand. Our brain has developed over millions of years, beginning with an instinctive, primitive mind, which we refer to as the Reptilian brain. This has to do with arousal and our sexual and other drives. And then came our middle brain, sitting nicely on top of our reptilian brain. This part of the brain is often referred to as the Paleomammalian brain or Limbic system. This part of the brain quickly developed over time to allow us to learn, remember and become emotional. And finally comes the mammalian brain or Neocortex, our highest layer, the top layer, seated nicely on the paleomammalian system. We evolved this part of our brain to experience conscious thought, self-awareness, and language and so on. All three of these layers do amazing things, they are connected in some ways and in other ways they are not. They communicate with one another constantly, making necessary alterations and changes where necessary, and at other times, they work independently of each other. They are also ever evolving, changing, and not set in concrete. They are elastic and flexible and can repair, change, and do many remarkable things that we are only now beginning to realize. Thanks to neuroscience and technological advances, we are getting to this understanding at a quicker rate than our predecessors could ever have imagined.

I would also like to add here that many of my clients often refer to 'people' as having a negative impact on their well-being. In other words, *my boss drives me crazy,* or *my partner is stressing me out!* People truly believe that other individuals (or external factors) cause them stress. But in fact, everything controls us from the inside. It has zero to do with stressful people, a demanding boss, or outside influences. It is the way we interpret those situations that counts. Welcome to Neuroscience. By understanding how our brains work, we will be in a better position to manage our emotions and behaviour.

Neuroscientists and Neurobiologists will also consider those people who present with neurological or psychiatric disorders. They will focus on behaviour, cognitive functions, and cellular communication networks, to assess the biological part of the emotional brain.

The scientific study of the neural system has increased significantly over the last twenty years or so, principally in the fields of molecular biology and computational skills. Advanced brain screening technology such as the latest Functional Magnetic Resonance Imaging (fMRI), Electroencephalogram (EEG) and Event-related Potentials (ERPs), Positron Emission Tomography (PET) and CT scans have allowed neurobiologists to study the nervous system in much more detail than ever before. They have observed its structure, how the brain is wired, how it operates, how it malfunctions and how it can be defined or exchanged. Neuroscientists have become experts on the brain and can understand in large detail the complex processes taking place in the nervous system, as well as the complex nature of the billions of tiny cells that work inside this organization. These brain cells are called neurons. And this is where Neuroplasticity comes in.

Neuroplasticity

The term *Neuro* relates to the brain or the nervous system. *Plasticity* refers to the ability of neurons to alter their reaction to what has gone on earlier. So, this means that neurons can change and be rejuvenated. They can be rewired and reprogrammed!

Neuroplasticity is essentially a term used to describe the brain's ability to renew and fix itself when needed. It states that the brain is not set in concrete or wired permanently, but rather, the brain is like plastic: you can mold and change and rebuild brain cells and neural connections to suit yourself in whatever way you wish. More importantly, neuroplasticity focuses on the brain's power to reorganize itself to forge new neural pathways as part of the brain's capacity to keep you functioning as normal. Neuroplasticity allows the neurons (nerve cells) to compensate for injury and disease and to adjust their activities in response to new situations and changes in the environment. It also tells us that we can alter neural activity in several non-invasive ways, such as the use of guided meditation, self-hypnosis, visualization and more, basically creating in your mind's eye the outcome you wish to achieve. Your thinking, and thoughts alone, can cause modifications in your brain, changing chemical messages to what you want them to broadcast. You can hack into your own brain, your neurons, to produce the results you want to see! This is truly amazing.

Neurons

A neuron is a nerve cell that sends chemical messages or nerve impulses to other neurons. Neurons process incoming data and then communicate that information through electrical and chemical signals at an exceedingly fast rate like that of the speed of light! Undamaged neurons can be altered. And this is where the broken neuron idea came from for this book. Broken neurons that are not physically damaged by injury or disease can be changed and sculptured in any fashion that you like. But also hold in mind that neurons are clever, and if they are permanently damaged, sometimes new neural networks will find another pathway to make up for the damaged cells. An example: an individual who loses their sight will soon fine-tune their other senses (hearing, smell, touch), as new neural networks take shape over time to compensate for the loss of vision. This is called Sensory Substitution. Also, as time moves on, new and more powerful neural networks will regenerate and grow around the damaged cells to offset the loss of sight by increasing the ability of the other senses.

The same theory applies when it comes to mental health and most of its disorders. With post-traumatic stress disorder, for instance, evidence tells us that the chemical levels in the brain change after the traumatic event, and in turn, so does the behaviour of the person. Are these chemical changes a direct link to shocked neurons after the traumatic experience? Let us quickly move back to Matthew's story. He suffered from PTSD. Were his neurons not firing and wiring happily together anymore? Did the shock of those traumas and the prolonged fear he experienced after those events cause his neurons to become broken? Was the speed of light transmissions between nerve cell and nerve cell harmed because of this? Were his neurons just temporarily broken or were they permanently damaged?

Matthew's neurons were not permanently damaged. He didn't suffer a physical injury, nor was he diagnosed with any organic abnormalities, so no everlasting damage was done. They were just momentarily broken, and this means that they were repairable. They were psychologically broken. They could be fixed with counselling and neuron therapy. Thus, if the shock and hurt he experienced consciously and unconsciously during those terrible events, and the aftermath of those negative experiences, led to his neurons breaking down, causing them to become weakened, resulting in his post-traumatic stress disorder diagnosis, the question is, can they return to normal? His neurons in that part of his brain were no longer happily firing and wiring together. They were not firing as they should. Because of this, Matthew continued to battle his uncontrollable feelings and wavering moods, because of his emotionally broken neurons. And yes, his fearful neurons could be repaired and returned to normal, as they were prior to those traumas.

Neurons are cells inside the neural organization that send data to other nerve cells, muscles, and glands. Most neurons have a cell body with dendrites and an axon. Dendrites extend from the cell body of the neuron to receive messages and then these messages are passed on down through the axon where they exit through the terminal branches (synaptic terminal) where they become neurotransmitters as they pass through the synaptic gap or synapse junction. And then the process is copied over and over—sending chemical messages from neuron to neuron, from dendrite down through the axon, and so on.

(See Diagram 1)

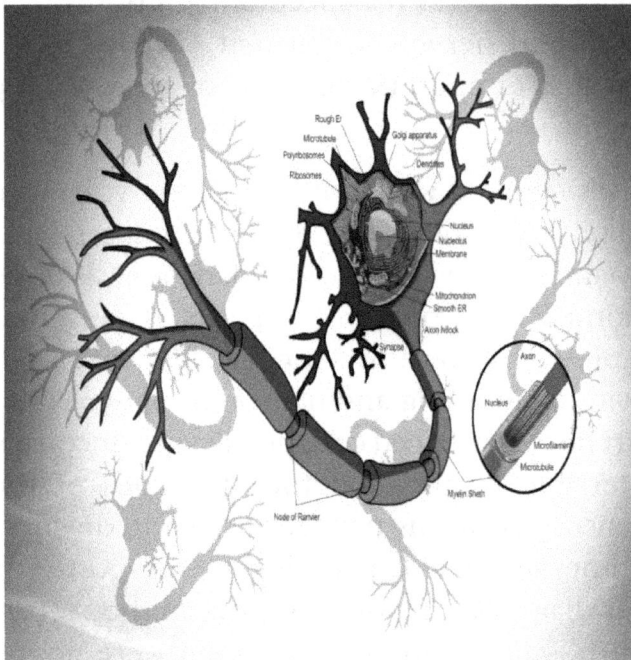

Diagram 1 is an image of the neuron and its description, including dendrites, axon, and terminal buttons. See enlarged version on page 57, this Chapter.

Neurotransmitters

Neurotransmitters are message carriers. They transmit messages between neurons in the brain (and the body) and are exchanged through the synapses between the neurons. They can be localized and can cause different outcomes for the person depending on their production, and whether they are increased or decreased. Researchers have found that depending on their production level, neurotransmitters can have a negative or positive impact on your emotional and physical well-being. Even environmental stress, with your permission (meaning the way you interpret this incoming data), can alter and change the overproduction or underproduction levels of your neurotransmitters. This means that external influences can affect the way your neurons fire and wire together. Internally, this can happen also. Meaning, your own negative thinking can have a hostile impact on your cells. External and internal influences can lead to your neurons becoming broken, therefore causing an adverse impact on the way they dispense the neurotransmitters (messages).

The most known neurotransmitters are serotonin and dopamine. GABA is another one I mention often with my clients because of its association with anxiety and relaxation. Gamma Amino Butyric Acid (GABA) is likewise related to poor or interrupted sleep. If this neurotransmitter is not functioning properly, anxiety in all its forms will peak and may yet thrive.

The Serotonin neurotransmitter is usually connected with cognitive and behavioural operations. It can affect the way a person thinks and feels depending on how this neurotransmitter works. At the same time, if this neurotransmitter is not functioning in good order, and is deficient in its production because the neuron is broken, then depression, feelings of isolation and disconnectedness, even apprehension and anxiety, may prevail.

Dopamine is another one of those neurotransmitters that we must pay close attention to. It needs to be working healthily to avoid harmful mental health outcomes. Dopamine is usually associated with joy, feeling great, and a sense of well-being and freedom. It also has to do with your motivation and enthusiasm. And as previously mentioned, if this neurotransmitter is not performing properly, then a lack or loss of interest will occur. The person will feel listless and will hold little or no energy or motivation to do much.

In the following chapter, we will examine Neuron Therapy, a term I coined to characterize this unique therapy. After years of research and, dare I say, trial and error, I finally perfected this therapy's method. I have witnessed continued success and the reversal of serious psychiatric disorders in clients who comprehended and understood the concept of this innovative therapy. This is an advanced and groundbreaking approach to managing your mental health, from the inside, on your terms.

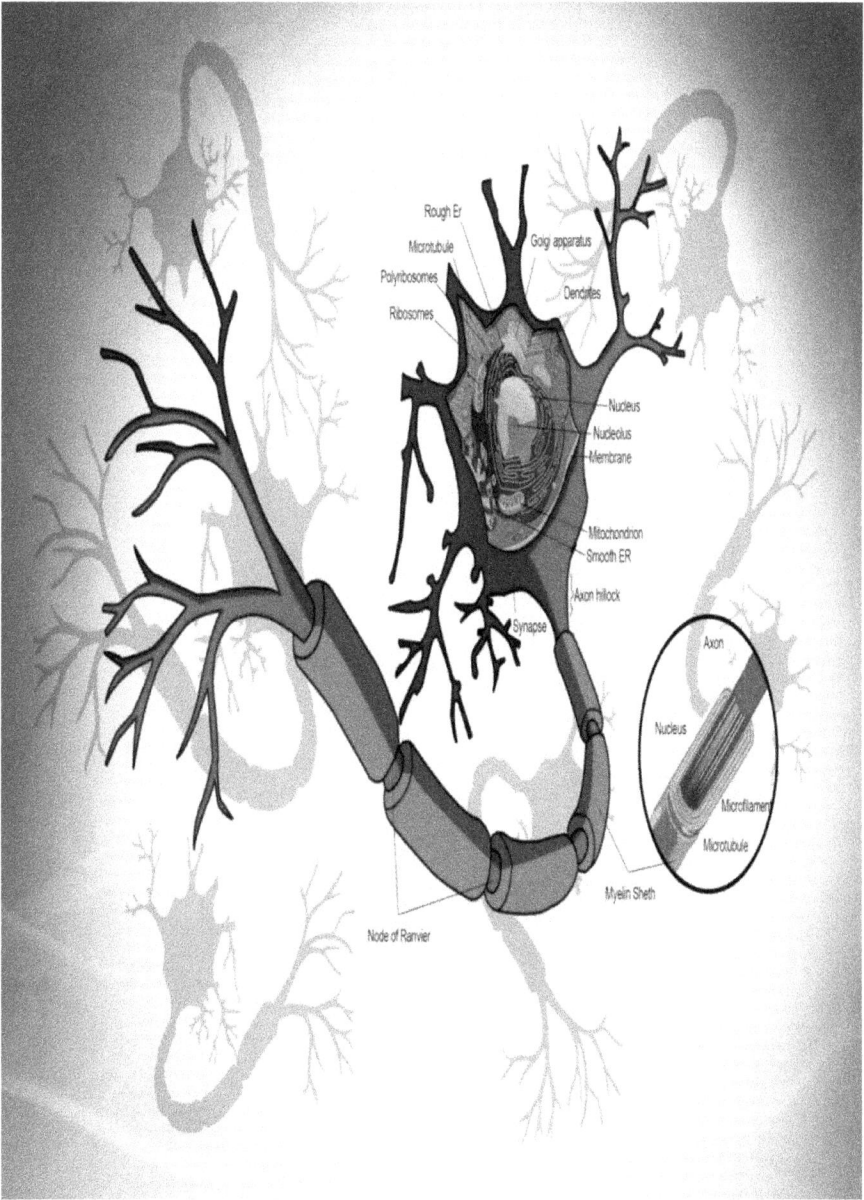

Rough Er
Microtubule
Polyribosomes
Ribosomes
Golg apparatus
Dendrites
Nucleus
Nucleolus
Membrane
Mitochondrion
Smooth ER
Axon hillock
Synapse
Axon
Nucleus
Microfilament
Microtubule
Myelin Sheth
Node of Ranvier

*Faith is taking the first step,
even if you don't see the
whole neural network.*

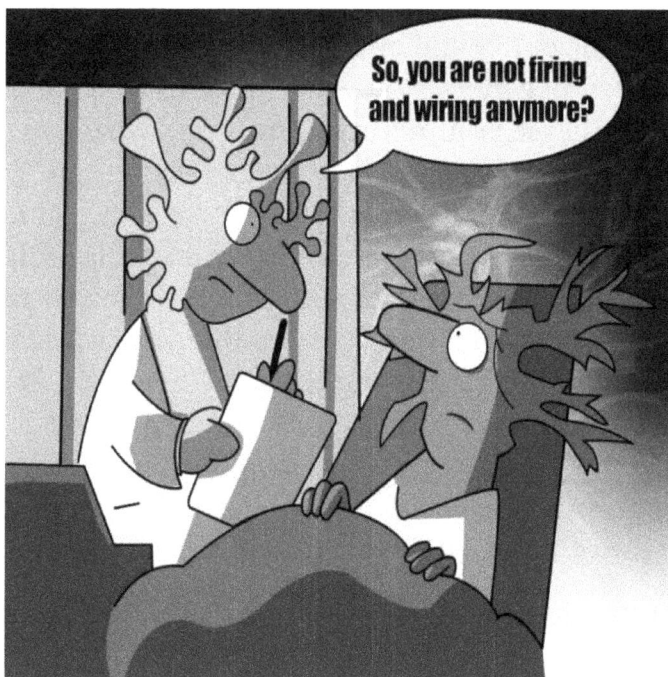

CHAPTER NINE:
Neuron Therapy

Back to the clients

This is a brief introduction to Neuron Therapy

Neuron Therapy is a technique that I created many years ago. Visualization and other forms of guided mental imagery are used to access the inner workings of your mind, particularly your neurons and neural networks, to gain control over these brain cells. This can usually be achieved by using your mind as a vessel to access your brain, like a ship sailing the ocean. The ship being your mind and the ocean being your brain. You are required to picture or imagine yourself shrinking into a microscopic entity and appearing in your brain, in your neural kingdom. Once there, you will be able to see your entire neural network and see your neurons firing and wiring as they should. It will no doubt be a sight (and feeling) to behold. You will need to use your imagination and visualize a world of neurons, and believe they are real, while in that minuscule world. Use your imagination to bring about intention, intention to create and fix and bring about a positive outcome. And while deep in your mind imagining your neural world, you will create energy around what you are doing. And where there is energy, there is healing. There is no right or wrong method here. Put simply, where attention goes, energy follows. Even wishful thinking will create change on the cellular level!

The aim of neuron therapy is to do the work from that perspective, in microscopic form, from a quantum viewpoint, using your intention and energy to fix your cells. The client is instructed to go about looking for 'broken' neurons and fixing them as they go along. The method here is whatever you wish that method to be, or what will work for you. Each client may use a different approach to make these inner changes.

I think it would be easier to introduce neuron therapy as you read the stories of the clients listed in this book. You will read for yourself how I introduced neuron therapy into their respective treatment plans and the many approaches that can be used to access your neural territory. It is all about going within to make changes that are so often reflected on the outside.

Briefly, let us revisit Cynthia's story. Remember, she was concerned that the many changes in her job role were having a negative impact on her emotions, causing apprehension, and making her stress flare up. I also noted that she was having significant challenges with cultural differences and being assertive in the workplace.

Cynthia originally underwent regular counselling sessions using evidence-based interventions and skills training to help her cope more fittingly with her situation. She struggled at first and even considered medication to help, but this went against her values as a health-minded person. Taking medication would also confirm to her that she was indeed sick, as she often reminded me. Cynthia was secretly ashamed to be in counselling and believed that only sick people should visit me. Her troubles were just work and stress and she always apologized for holding up my time, as she puts it, when she came for her consultations.

When I introduced neuron therapy into her counselling sessions, Cynthia had difficulties understanding this idea at first. But when we externalized her neurons and individualized them, she understood almost immediately. Cynthia's unique worldview had created similar neurons (mirror neurons) and over the years, she reinforced them unknowingly, surrounding herself with like-minded people, eventually seeing that she had lost her power over her neurons and that they were now in the driver's seat, controlling not only her thoughts and emotions but also her behaviour. Cynthia had lost her ability to be flexible and independent, she had painted herself into a neurotic corner, all because of her hectic, unpredictable, and ever-increasing workload.

For those who are unfamiliar with the term mirror neurons, it simply means 'mirroring' the behaviour or actions of others. In Cynthia's case, she was mirroring (mimicking) what she believed her employers wanted from her, unaware that there were other options and other ways of doing her job. She tried imitating her high-flying colleagues in the corporate world and worked 24 hours a day to get their approval, without any focus on work-life balance or the effects this had on her mind and body. And then she ended up in counselling.

Over the years, Cynthia had strengthened some of her brain neurons and weakened others, unknowingly, through everyday living. Her healthy neurons were working well, firing, and wiring happily together, glowing. Unfortunately, her broken neurons were sluggish, not wiring and firing properly anymore, looking dull and tired. Not glowing. These broken neurons were sending signals to the outside, attempting to find the owner's attention. And the only way they knew how to get the owner's attention, was to turn on the fight and flight response survival system. This is when apprehension and stress are revealed physically, a direct call for help from broken neurons deep inside your head. These broken neurons were the cause of Cynthia's distress, and over time, they became weakened from her intensive workload. Also, Cynthia had altered her neurons over the years to fit in with her hectic and unsustainable lifestyle, reinforcing her unhelpful worldview and self-defeating behaviours, which in turn, sapped her central nervous system of vital energy, moving her whole body into incoherence and conflict with other biological systems.

Still, Cynthia believed that she had to feed all of herself to her work to be a dependable employee. These unrealistic thinking patterns also extended to her children and faithful acquaintances. She believed that she should work and work and never question her superiors, no matter how unreasonable they were or what they expected from her. Meanwhile, the silent (and sometimes loud) cries from her inner world were ignored. Cynthia's outer world mattered more.

As she continued her debilitating journey, Cynthia applied the same unworkable approach to her personal life, wanting to be there for everyone, all the time. She also worked long hours and did not get compensated for her regular overtime, often missing important family occasions. Cynthia did for others what others did not do for her. She also told me that she took four days off work when her mother passed away, as she had to attend the funeral in China, leaving on a Thursday night and returning the following Monday night. This was a flight between Sydney and Shanghai and back. Her explanation at the time, 'The manager would be angry if I took more time off to bury my mother.'

During her time in China, Cynthia received many calls from her work colleagues about work-related business. Not once did Cynthia think this was unfair or unreasonable, even though she was grieving. She returned quickly to work on her return and continued working those long and arduous hours, being there for everyone—without fail.

Cynthia did not have an assertive neuron to rely on. Her neurons were passive by nature, and they became that way from many years of programming. Her neurons were now broken, slaves to a faulty thinking process that was not favourable to Cynthia's emotional well-being. Her neurons were long overdue for an overhaul. They were in desperate need of seeing a counsellor. But can these neurons be repaired? Are they fixable? The simple answer is yes. Changes can be made. I will get back to her story a little later and share with you how Cynthia and I tackled her broken neurons and how she repaired them all by herself.

Think of young Ben when he first arrived with his parents. They were concerned about his attention deficit disorder (ADD) mentioned to him by several professionals. They were worried about his forgetfulness and not sustaining attention and losing things almost daily. His mother secretly told me that she had had many diagnoses or comments from professionals in the medical and teaching fields, speculating that Ben may have autism or oppositional defiant disorder related to attention deficit disorder. Ben's mother didn't know what to believe anymore, but after many months of taking her son from one appointment to another, the ADD verdict seemed to pop up more often than the other disorders. His age plays a significant role when it comes to working out what it is with Ben and his behaviours. Thus, Ben was now acting out and becoming belligerent and then crying hysterically. He was developing anxiety around his condition. He could feel and sense the fear in his parents, especially his mother. His parents were emotionally drained, to say the least, and his mother looked like she was going to burst into tears whenever we talked.

How can neuron therapy work here? Ben is young and for him to understand the intricate workings of his emotional mind, and brain cells would be a long shot, to say the least. But you know what? Children grasp the neuron discovery much quicker than adults, usually. I think children have not yet acquired a worldview about themselves. They do not hold a firm belief system about how things should be. So, looking at neurons is all part of growing up and nothing unusual to the child. It's simply part of therapy for them.

Many children identify with basic emotions. A happy neuron means happy. An angry neuron equals angry. Simple! In a conversational manner, it is simple, but the underlying biological and chemical conditions occurring within our brains are complicated, far too complicated to be explained here, and the aim with all of this is to keep things uncomplicated. I recall a wise individual once telling me, *the world is a simple place to live in; however, we complicate things and make the world a challenge to survive in.* So, a tip for you all, keep things simple! Life is really not that complicated.

We will arrive back to Ben and his baffling neurons later.

Let us look at Stephen's case now. If you remember, Stephen's mother dragged him to counselling because of his uncontrollable behaviour. He was just sixteen at the time. He was diagnosed with a generalized anxiety disorder with panic symptoms. He had also become aggressive and was abusive to nearly everyone who was close to him. His mother was at the end of her tether. She was also a single mother.

As usual and routine, a treatment plan was carried out and cognitive behavioural therapy and interpersonal therapy were all employed with various skills training. Stephen responded well to the reward system, seeing his achievements in real-time. Like many young people, neuron therapy was a norm for him. He held no thought that this was part of a novel and revolutionary science, and quickly embraced this plan of attack. Once he saw how his neurons worked for him, the more he saw how they influenced his thinking and behaviour. He found it fascinating that neurons controlled him and that they were so small, microscopic. The following were his words, and he was right. Referring to those neurons that he was experiencing trouble managing, he gave them nicknames, calling them 'micro shits'.

Changing pace here, let us look at Patrick's story quickly. He was suffering with severe depression and had lost the will to live. He was a tortured man and suffered daily with his condition. He could not feel inner contentment or joy anymore. Patrick had seen many counsellors over the years, but he was ambivalent with his responses about the outcomes of those sessions, stating that some helped him for a short while, and then reporting later that no one had helped him. He describes his situation as always returning to his status quo position, which he calls a dark and lonely place and the only company he has there is the ever-lurking black dog, watching him with persecuting eyes, tempting him to just give up and stop wrestling with life.

Patrick's neurons were not just ruined, but they had abandoned their positions. Where on earth did his neurons go? Usually, broken neurons are still struggling along, but they are in place, as we say. Meaning, they should be where they are supposed to be. First, we had to find them, and this was an ordeal, but Patrick gave me the benefit of the doubt because, if you remember, he told me that I was flogging a dead horse when it came to supporting him. He told me that since I had faith in him, he will try one more time to manage his low mood, thus showing some enthusiasm to find his missing depressed neurons. Did we end up finding them? Maybe, but let us move on to the next client, as all will be revealed later.

Jacquie was in her late thirties and came to me out of despair. She had found that I could assist her with personal development, and she desired to 'fix' herself before her big Fortieth birthday, as she put it. Jacquie had given up on love. She told me that she had come to terms with her plight and that she was starting to get herself comfy and give up on ever finding a suitable partner. Sadly, she confessed that growing pot plants and investing in a kitten or puppy, or both, sounded promising in terms of living a single life. I intervened and reminded her that life was not that bleak. I also pointed to the charcoal drawing she had framed and given to me to hang in my waiting room. Jacquie was quite gifted, creating near masterpieces with her pencil sketches and charcoal drawings. She told me that her dream was to one day sell her work online, but for now, she had bigger fish to fry, as she put it.

If you can remember, Jacquie was unlucky in love and had many relationships over the years, but they ended sooner than she wished. She fondly talked about her first love when she was eighteen. The relationship lasted about five years and she was happy. She believed that he was her perfect match. Sadly, he went off to study at university in another state and left Sydney. Their relationship ended shortly after. She told me that since her first relationship, she has never been in a relationship longer than about three months or so. She was at a loss about why this was happening to her and why she couldn't find a long-term boyfriend. At first, she blamed the men. She told me the men she dated became inconsistent soon after, telling lies and not committing to the relationship. Then she added that initially, they were altogether marvellous, loving, and attentive, but then things changed, and they would get distant and suspicious, and their personalities would change. Are all men like that? Aren't men interested in long-term committed relationships anymore? Jacquie was confused and resentful.

When introduced to neuron therapy, Jacquie raised her professional eyebrows. She asked me if I were crazy and how would that fix her relationship problems? After all, men are out there in the real world, not swimming around in her head. However, Jacquie was desperate. She was hoping for a miracle remedy. She was hoping that I would take that magic wand out of my desk drawer and wave it over her head and presto! A man, perfect in every way. But to no avail. We had to perform the hard work together. We had to dig deep and get our hands dirty. We had to find those elusive neurons that shied away from the male of the species. We had to ask those neurons directly what the hell was going on, and why were they sabotaging Jacquie's relationships with potential partners? And do you know what? They ended up telling us. This was when Jacquie collapsed in a heap on my floor. The revealing and confronting information was the last thing Jacquie wanted to hear. So, what information came forward? You'd probably be surprised. Don't worry, I will be returning to this case later. But for now, I need to move on to Matthew's section.

Remember that phrase, 'stuck in the moment of horror'? That was Matthew's story. Post-Traumatic Stress Disorder (PTSD) is a soul-destroying disorder, according to Matthew. PTSD is one of the anxiety disorders and can often trigger other mental illnesses if not managed suitably.

Matthew went along with neuron therapy without any fuss. He was defeated and had nothing more to lose, or hardly any energy to challenge me with what I was suggesting. He didn't even lift an eyebrow when I mentioned going inside to fix and heal broken neurons. He simply looked at me with a straight face, and I wondered what was running through his intellect as he sat there, deadpan. And when I mentioned, perhaps trying the Grape process, tears welled up in his eyes. Perhaps he was thinking that maybe I had finally gone mad and that his last hope had just lost the plot altogether. Or, he may have been thinking that he had finally reached the end of his road of pain, and this was the final straw, allegorically speaking. Nevertheless, this is the nature of these disorders, an uncontrollable show of emotions at times, especially becoming fearful and/or crying for no obvious cause.

How will neuron therapy help this man recover and get his life back? His case is as interesting as all the cases mentioned in this book. I will come back to his story a little later, as I am trying to give brief summarizations so you can better understand how neuron therapy works when it comes to the individuals presented in this book.

Cassandra is the 'yo-yo' person who sadly talked about her weight problem. Many can probably relate to her frustrations when she said it was like putting on a few kilos after drinking a small glass of water. She often questioned, she told me, when out and about and watching what she refers to as skinny people stuffing their faces with the most ghastly of foods, and yet they remained bone thin. Sarcastically and bitterly, Cassandra referred to those people as lollipops, suggesting that they were so sparse, their heads appeared much larger than their physical structure, from the neck down. She would then apologize for making such cattish statements and then get teary.

Cassandra had many issues she needed to address, from trying to manage her binge eating to working out what she wanted to do with her life in terms of career and friends. She also wrestled with continuing family conflicts between her parents and fearing the loss of her close friends. 'Everything has changed since I left high school. I hardly see any of my friends anymore', she exclaimed. University life was also challenging for her, and she found it increasingly difficult to keep up with studies and assignments, maintaining new friendships and managing her family problems.

When introduced to neuron therapy, Cassandra became excited. She enjoyed the mystical theme. She had often seen psychics and numerologists about her circumstances, and she had read magazines to do with her star sign. Cassandra wanted to know more and sat up straight in the session, and I remembered pointing out to her then, that this was the most animated I'd ever seen her in our sessions together. Like a duck to water, Cassandra not only embraced neuron therapy but excelled!

Over the next chapters, I will be showing you, the reader, how neuron therapy works, and how you can also manage your own mental health concerns from this perspective. Also, think of what I stated at the start of this book that not all people will profit from this therapy or approach. As with everything, even evidence-based therapies, not everyone will respond as we would wish them to.

CHAPTER TEN:
Metaphysical and Quantum Therapy

Your Brain does not only perform at the physical level.

This is about understanding your *physical* and *non-local* brain.

Going on the inside to fix the outside.

Metaphysical and Quantum Therapy (MQT) is a method of intentionally and visually exploring your neurons and making positive changes from the inside, according to your plans. This is another therapy I created a few years back, and it is a direct extension of neuron therapy. Evidence tells us that engaging in physical activities and learning by memorizing and through repetitive activities can bring about inner changes. It is like visualization, guided imagery, counselling, self-hypnosis and so on. Essentially, it means the more you practice something, the more expert you will become in that activity or subject. The same goes for changing thinking patterns and behaviour.

Let's briefly examine the metaphysical aspect. Metaphysical typically refers to something that is unseen, esoteric, spiritual, supernatural, mystical, abstract, and cannot be understood or evaluated from a scientific or practical standpoint. It entails having faith in something that cannot necessarily be verified through 'physical' means. Perhaps, like karma. Many believe in karma, but when asked for proof, they appear dumbfounded. However, they believe, nonetheless.

Quantum mechanics or Quantum physics is a rather new science, well, it's been around for over a hundred years, but we are still trying to understand the science behind it. So, research continues. Quantum Mechanics, or Quantum Physics or Theory, is a subdivision of natural philosophy that deals with physical phenomena on molecular, atomic, nuclear, subatomic, and even on smaller microscopic levels. Many call this science the 'spooky science', for a good reason. They say physicists were baffled in the past (and even today!) when viewing atoms and tiny particles under the microscope, only to find, to their amazement, that these tiny particles would change properties depending on who was watching. Wait, there's more. These atoms can exist in two spaces at one time! And they appear to be linked invisibly to each other, a term called entanglement; they can communicate or react instantaneously with the other, no matter how far apart they are and no matter what the distance. It is like they are connected psychically, as no physical links between them are present.

The hypothesis goes that metaphysical and quantum therapy (MQT) can be applied to focus attention on our brain cells to bring about changes we seek, impacting profoundly on the electromagnetic field surrounding each of our billions of cells and our body as a whole. Some call this Neuro-hacking. Changing or fixing redundant thinking patterns and behaviours from within.

Mainstream therapies are standard practice and usually work well, but sometimes we need to go a little further when these approaches do not work for the client. By incorporating MQT into the client's treatment plan, the client will need to memorize how to zero in on brain cells and other microscopic nerve cells, on a spiritual and psychic level. They can accomplish this through self-hypnosis or visualization techniques. Others again prefer the power of prayer. Praying for outcomes you desire.

Guided imagery or visualization techniques are often used in my practice, and this is when you need to think like the quantum entanglement theory, where you try to influence and alter your broken neurons by observation, sending your healing energies to the damaged neuron, persuading those neurons to start wiring and firing again as they should. The neurons and their networks need to light up; they need to glow and beam. The brighter they are, the healthier you are. You should be able to see all of this in your quantum and metaphysical microstate because you have withered down to the cellular level and are in full view of your neurons and neural nets. Now that you are there, the work needs to be done, from the inside, and not with physical hands, but with the power of will and intention. Remember, where attention goes, energy flows. And energy carries messages. Just like spooky quantum physics. By mere observation, you are causing energy to affect the object you are observing, hence different outcomes for different people, as they are sending different energy to the same object by focusing their individual attention on the object or thing they wish to change. Now bring in the metaphysical side of things, and you have a potent tool to make inner changes to neurons and their neural networks from a spiritual perspective, and on a minuscule level. The work you are doing is well outside the domain of scientific knowledge, but so is MQT and Neuron Therapy, for now. Not everything is based on tangible matter; an unknown spiritual realm is also in play.

Is Part of our Brain Non-Locally Based?

The more I research this area the more my brain aches. Nothing makes sense in the real, concrete world, but on a metaphysical level or quantum level, it surprisingly does. So sometimes one needs to tread outside the bubble of physical life and look the unseen world directly in its eye. In other words, meet your neurons in person, not as a being of matter, but as an entity of energy!

Scientists tell us that our brain is a biochemical and bioelectric system. Like a biological computer or command centre. But the brain is much more than that. Scientists don't tell us about other functions of the brain, such as where all the vast, complex, and miraculous information is stored. Perhaps they don't know. They also don't tell us how the brain can send and receive messages in a flash, like the speed of light, and do all these things simultaneously and instantaneously, day in and day out, until we die. Even more incredible, the electrical messages are not just racing along chemical 'physical' routes, but also sending messages across space and time from one cellular bit to another without any physical connections to the other, as if by magic, or some scientists speculate, telepathically. No hard wiring needed! This is precisely how quantum physics works. And this is how our neurons work also. They are constantly receiving and sending messages from one another by means of neurotransmitters and through other means that we are yet to understand. They seem to anticipate and react before becoming consciously aware as if operating 'faster' than physical time itself. They are broadcasting messages from here to there and everywhere—all at one time, and in a split second. And when our neurons are broken, or not working as they should, they slow down into our perception of reality and physical time. This is when we can intervene. This is when we can do the repair job from the inside, through willpower, prayer, visualization, guided imagery, wishful thinking and using symbolism to influence changes on the inside.

In a nutshell, some scientists now think that our brain is not merely a physical organ working like a mechanical machine, but a highly organized and yet to be understood complex system, capable of impossible and invisible tasks that we are just now finding out. There also appears to be an aspect of the brain that has a non-local component, a paranormal function. There is a portion of our mind that is intuitive and seems to be connected to the past and future. I, and others in this field, propose that this piece of our mind is responsible for those gut feelings and instincts about events seemingly unperceivable through our normal physical senses. And where does consciousness fit in? Is consciousness found in our physical brain or is it also non-local, being 'out there', somewhere? This is the question that has so long vexed scientists and philosophers. Traditionally, the scientific community has tried to define consciousness as the product of brain activity. But growing evidence supports the idea that consciousness goes far beyond the physical workings of the brain. They further hypothesize that consciousness goes *outside* our physical selves.

The evidence seems to be there, and the results speak for themselves. Many individuals from diverse backgrounds report that their mind (consciousness) was still present even when their bodies showed no signs of life. They were clinically dead but had an awareness of what was going on around them, before returning to their body when brought back to life. From merely a scientific point of opinion, however, this cannot be proved directly, yet. Furthermore, I can exclusively support these findings, as the supernatural experiences reported to me on frequent occasions by many of my clients, from various backgrounds and ages, and over many years, eerily confirm the above presumptions.

Just like in quantum physics, there are many aspects that can't be explained about our brain, but they exist. Once we have the technology and more modern information processing systems, the non-local part of our brains will be revealed, and this will change everything. Besides MQT and Neuron Therapy, I believe the field of psychology will change to something new, and all psychological interventions will take place from the inside, by the client themselves, rather than sitting in a room listening to guidance from an extraneous source.

Finally, I mentioned symbolism earlier. Many of my clients have used symbolism to help them manage their neurons, just like counselling and other methods. Symbolism can mean many things to different people. It can be used as a figure of speech where a person or object has another meaning other than its literal meaning. An example: life is a roller coaster (meaning that life will have its ups and downs) or the black dog won't let me go (meaning the individual is suffering with depression). Symbolism can also be used in colours: white usually represents love and purity; black usually represents death and evil; red may be associated with passion and danger and so on. So, if you see a picture of a black menacing dog standing over a man in a foetal position on the floor, with a huge teardrop beside the man, it instantly gives you the message. This is symbolism at its best. It is the quintessential picture worth a thousand words.

Those individuals using symbolism to enter their neuron kingdom will develop stories to create symbols and fantasy tools to help them along the way. They may visualize holding on to a particular object that holds meaning for them; a meaningful item given to them by their grandfather or mother, such as a war medal or a piece of jewellery handed down through the ages, or perhaps a piece of garment or a picture of someone special. These items may symbolize strength and courage for that person, and they will take the item with them on their journey while trying to make contact directly with their neurons. It is like a protection object, a tool to give them inner strength and the ability to face the hidden demons that may be lurking at the gates of their microscopic world. Some people may use a ladder to rise up, or maybe a bridge they need to traverse over to enter that state of intellect. Some will play mystical music, drums thumping in the backdrop, a tambourine sounding, or messing up a flute. There is a particular process the individual needs to follow to gain entry.

The cluster of grapes idea has become the most common method employed by my clients to enter the neuron realm. Imagine or picture a healthy swollen bunch of ripened purple-black, luscious grapes, free of blemishes or insects. It looks delicious and flawless, perfect in every way. Now imagine the bunch of grapes is your neurons and neural networks. Each individual grape in the bunch is a neuron. Each neuron is connected to your emotions and behaviour. If the bunch of grapes is healthy and playing well, they will be glowing with white illumination. They will be working happily together and without any troubles. However, what if some of the neurons are broken? Damaged in some fashion? Some of the grapes or neurons on the bunch are not working or playing anymore? They are fused, not glowing any longer. These neurons will affect the whole neural network, and this is when your clever brain and body begin to display warning signals to its owner in the way of anxiety, depression, anger and so on. Those are the gut feelings you feel when something may be amiss. Broken neurons that are not working as they should, can cause a negative impact on your emotions and behaviour if left untreated. And as their health deteriorates, they will scream out for help by displaying physical symptoms to get your attention.

Those bunches of grapes (or neurons and their networks) not working effectively will have individual grapes switched off, indicating that the grape is broken. Symbolically speaking, that is why you have entered this world, to fix those individual grapes and encourage them to start working again, glowing brightly, as they fire together and wire together, as they should. The individual needs to go from one grape (neuron) to another and ensure that they are glowing and shining simultaneously, throwing forth a healthy radiance. All of this will be taking place in your mind as you visualize yourself there, in energy form, willing and envisioning those neurons to resume normal operation once again. The power of the mind should not be underestimated. By merely believing that a change is occurring, your brain and neural networks will begin to produce these physical changes within the brain, thereby producing the results you have programmed by thought and will power alone.

Metaphysical and Quantum Therapy, and Neuron Therapy adopts this approach, where we incorporate visualization and intention techniques to establish contact with broken neurons. Once there, we use our mental energy to create the necessary changes that are required.

As you read on, you will discover how these revolutionary therapies can assist one's mental health. I presume it may also make more sense as we relate this therapy to the specific cases I will now describe in detail.

CHAPTER ELEVEN:
Cynthia:
How the Ship Helped Me

Going inside to fix the outside

Following consistent sessions with me, Cynthia eventually grasped the concept of counselling. She initially found therapy intimidating and foreign. She could not comprehend the rationale behind counselling and, more specifically, caring for her own wants and needs. She had a profound sense that her purpose on earth was to facilitate and aid others. This was the position she held in life. She was destined to be a team player, a loyal and diligent employee, unquestioning and constantly striving. This was Cynthia's worldview, and it directly contradicted counselling. After she got over her initial shock about what was expected of her in therapy, she began to challenge her belief system of how she saw the world. She realized that by being the way she was, she was in fact making herself mentally sick. She wanted to be there for her children and wanted to be around to see them marry, eventually having children themselves. This was the motivator for Cynthia to make those necessary psychological changes.

Cynthia was not helped by cognitive therapy or the behavioural component of therapy. She found that approach to be too difficult. She was unable to restructure her thought patterns using rational thought because, according to her, it was against her values and made no sense to her. However, she reacted well to the skills training and even wanted to learn more about parenting skills and conversational training. She said that she had always found communication a challenge, especially with new people and after the initial touch and greet. She told me she ran out of things to say, and then that was that. Ironically, she told me she found most people boring, however, she was quick to remind me that she was tiring as well!

As you may know by now, neuron therapy is an approach where you use visualization and other forms of mental imagery to access the inner workings of your brain, with the aim of contacting your neurons and brain cells. This can be accomplished by using your preferred method of guided visualization, or self-hypnosis or creative thinking, whatever you feel comfortable with. Many of my previous clients like the analogy of using the mind as the vessel to access their brain; like a ship sailing across the sea; the ship being your mind and the ocean being your brain. In neuron therapy, the mind and brain are two different things, they are not one and the same. Your brain is that physical organ that sits inside your head, whereas the mind is that part that sits here, there, and everywhere. As mentioned earlier, some scientists theorize that your mind (or part of it) may be non-local, and from what I have garnered over the years, this theory makes sense. So, getting back to Cynthia, she needed to use her mind to gain access to her brain. Her mind had the keys to unlock the physical components of her brain.

Cynthia did not wish to use symbolism or to have a protector item with her. She was ready to confront her inner kingdom as herself with no props or weapons. I reminded her of her Other Self, a potentially provocative aspect of herself, her polar opposite, her cosmic self, which was observing and watching.

Each of us is guided by two energies or forces: our conscious, rational side that responds to external stimuli, and our unconscious, which is governed by internal causes. When necessary, both parties can cross over to the other side and communicate with each other, but for the most part, they remain on their respective sides of the psychological fence. Further, they also perform independently from each other. Therefore, for Cynthia to obtain admission, she must be conscious of her two selves and overcome them to contact her neurons. Generally, my clients use rational and practical methods to bypass the conscious intellect, as they normally have direct access to this portion of their brain. Yet, they have all kinds of problems communicating directly with their unconscious mind, for the simple fact, it's unconscious. This is where self-hypnosis and visualization play their role. Prayer and mantras and music may also aid in establishing contact. As many may know, instinct and intuition are the unconscious mind's vernacular. Listen inwardly, and you will hear it. To obtain access, an open heart is required. You must give up all your judgements. To establish contact, you must abandon critical thinking and presumptions. You must perceive and experience its cosmic language while turning off your conscious mind to enter. You must have faith in both of your minds, but particularly your unknown mind, your unconscious. Accept the undiscovered psyche. I also mentioned an additional aspect of your unconsciousness earlier. This unknown and elusive entity is referred to as one's 'Other Self.' This other unknown aspect of yourself is your spiritual self. A portion of you that is unrestricted by your physical body.

From the perspective of the conscious mind and using the ship on the ocean as a metaphor, this is how we know things to be. You stand firmly on deck as the ship sails across the ocean, as you move forward to eventually reach land. All physical and logical steps are taken here. However, from an unconscious point of view, you are no longer standing firmly on the ship, but rather flying high above it and have long since reached land! Nothing physical or rational here. This is how your unconscious mind works. The physical principles of nature do not apply in the quantum or neuron world. Therefore, what you believe or create in this magical world will manifest and influence change at the cellular level. Your thoughts and beliefs cause an inner transformation that will be reflected on the outside as well.

Cynthia employed her 'Other Self' to contact her neurons. To accomplish this, she had to first learn how to levitate above her ship instead of standing on deck. She was required to silence her conscious mind, her usual passive self. She had to detach herself from her physical limitations and become fearless and independent by relying on her imagination and mental strength. She had to trust and accept what was coming. She had to look the nothingness in the face with courage and conviction. She needed to overcome her anxieties. And once she accomplished this, the void would transform into something that she would recognize. A tranquil location in which her intangible Other Self resides.

After a while, Cynthia finally reached her neuron world with the help of enchanting and traditional Chinese music to help her along the way. Cynthia imagined, while in a profound state of meditation, a city of glowing neurons functioning, firing, and wiring as they should. According to her descriptions, it was a magnificently luminous scene. Everyone will approach and describe their neuron world differently, but all will portray the same underlying representation. Cynthia was no longer in her physical body; she had effectively escaped the physical dimension and could now move at the speed of light. And as she flew over her enchanted inner world of microscopic nerve cells, despite being minuscule herself, she could detect which direction to head. In the quantum world, however, anything is conceivable. This is where magic lingers. The damaged neurons of Cynthia, like infants, were crying out for their mother. They led Cynthia directly to themselves. And Cynthia intuitively knew exactly where they were. As she neared, the feeble lights revealed their location. They were not shining as brightly as they should. They were sick and broken. At last, they gasped; our mother had come home to save us.

Did you notice Cynthia's description of her microscopic world? The connotation here is that of a mother rescuing her babies. This was Cynthia's worldview, and this allowed her to gain entry and fix what needed to be fixed. Using the mother and the baby analogy worked for Cynthia as she was a mother herself. I remember Andrew, another one of my clients not mentioned in this book; he was fascinated by surfboards and skateboards and could not live without them. Hence, you can imagine how (and on what) this young man would enter his neuron world.

When contacting your neuron world, it is sometimes necessary to leave and return to the tangible and physical world to simulate how you will repair your broken neurons in the quantum world. Here, preparation comes into play. First, you must determine the nature of the problem; then, you must devise a solution to that problem. You must also be specific, addressing one problem and one step at a time. As a result of her cultural differences and lack of self-advocacy, Cynthia's anxiety and tension were caused by faulty thought patterns. This repeated action affected a subset of her neurons.

Cynthia had become a workaholic over the years, disregarding other aspects of her emotional health. Her existence had become devoid of recreation. Her entire universe consisted of work, and this was the most significant aspect of her existence. Because we are comprised of numerous components, each should be honoured and respected. Work is only one aspect, as are recreation and enjoyment. Relationships and intimacy, as well as physical activity and health, are two others. And there are many more aspects of who we are. Without recreation, Cynthia's neurons have no voice. And when they have no voice, they eventually shut down and break.

So, what should Cynthia do to repair her neurons? She required a solid plan. She needed to be specific about the first task she would undertake. Anxiety is a disorder predicated on fear, and her fears kept her in her flawed mindset. She had the false belief that her existence consisted entirely of work. And if she did not give of herself more than one hundred percent, twenty-four hours a day, then she would be a bad person and judged accordingly. Her fear here was that she would be rejected by not only her employer but by society as well. Her broken neurons were broken because they were swollen with the energy of rejection. The adjoining neurons were damaged because they had guilt written all over them. And don't forget the humiliation neurons, withering away in the corner; unloved, unvalued, and out of sight, oozing with the fear of being shamed.

Cynthia erupted into tears when she met her neurons one by one and witnessed firsthand, from a neural network perspective, what was happening at the cellular level. She could not comprehend the extent of the micro-level destruction. How could she continue to tolerate this? Poor neurons! Her babies! Neglected!

To repair her damaged neurons, rejuvenate them, or, in extreme cases, construct an entirely new neural network around them, she needed a detailed plan with new codes. In addition, Cynthia had to reassure her neurons by sending visual transmissions and images of love and forgiveness, as well as imprinting her new codes with rational information, so that the defective codes and self-defeating information could be expunged or made less prevalent.

The new set of rules would be based on her own requirements and desires; she would replace them with a healthy and beneficial energy that would help her neurons reconnect and fire normally once more. Her new protocol would be that she would come first. Health is the most essential aspect of life. Her profession is no longer her top priority. These new codes would be anxiety-reduction techniques. The purpose of these new codes will be to challenge her old, flawed thought patterns and self-defeating behaviours, replacing them with rational and helpful thought patterns and actions.

Cynthia realized that by altering her internal perspective of herself and the world, this would be reflected externally as well. Remember, the 'outside' will not change your interior thoughts and actions. Only you can, from the inside. By making these interior changes and acting on them, Cynthia not only made rapid progress in managing her anxiety and resentment, but she also became a more spontaneous and content individual. And at last, her daughters and her neurons were thrilled to have their mother back.

Neuron therapy was effective for Cynthia, as were other approaches, but this woman required neuron therapy to comprehend what was going on with her on a deeper level. She also realized that she had to continue checking on her neural world to ensure that everything was in order. By relapsing or reverting to old thought patterns, her neurons would once again become damaged, and her anxiety would return. Therefore, ongoing maintenance was required.

Intriguingly, everyone has a unique description of their neural world, and Cynthia described hers as resembling Shanghai at night as seen from above, with countless dazzling lights.

CHAPTER TWELVE:
Ben:
How Soccer Helped Me

Recapping young Ben's story, he was the little boy that his parents brought to my rooms because of his attention deficit disorder diagnosis. Many in my field are reluctant to render a one-hundred percent diagnosis of this disorder because we don't know a lot about it; only that treating its symptoms usually works. Many researchers in this area speculate that there may be underlying concerns, whether that is biological, emotional, or psychological and that these symptoms may be related to other childhood disorders. It may also be something different, something that we are yet to discover. But we have seen some positive results from therapy and medication, and we say to ourselves, at least that is working. But as you know, what is right for the goose may not necessarily be right for the gander. Or what is good for little Eddy may not be good for little Adam.

Ben's circumstance was complex. The therapy was partially effective, and he responded more to my relationship with him than to the tools I taught him. Ben enjoyed attending his sessions and included me as a member of his extended family, presenting me with his school achievements and anticipating telling me about his accomplishments. In a therapeutic relationship between a client and a counsellor, rapport is crucial, and we had accomplished this in Ben's sessions. His parents were relieved that he was attending therapy, as he previously refused to see a counsellor.

After discontinuing therapy at one point, Ben relapsed and was required to resume his sessions. Ben had previously seen several clinicians and therapists, and I was the last one he saw. In terms of regulating his emotions, he had made significant strides and settled down. His academics also improved, and his teacher noted a marked improvement in his disposition and demeanour.

So, against my wishes, his parents made the decision for him to cease all counselling. They informed me that they and young Ben had endured enough inconvenience due to their obligation to attend appointments. Perhaps he was simply going through a phase. That was their opinion. Unfortunately, this was not the situation. A few weeks later, Ben's mother received an urgent phone call from his school informing her of her worst fears. A message no parent wishes to receive. Ben had attempted self-harm before fleeing the school and vanishing down the road. His horrified and distraught mother rushed to the school to learn what had happened to her son.

After an altercation during recess with other boys, it was clear that Ben had had enough. What transpired during their morning break and what was said between them is largely unknown. Ben later explained to me that he was taunted and subsequently ran to the rear of the schoolyard towards the oval and the out-of-bounds bush area. He stumbled upon some broken glass in the dirt, and in a fit of rage, he seized it and stabbed himself in the side of his stomach, slicing his hand and fingers in the process. It was determined that his injuries were not life-threatening.

He did not attend a hospital, nor did he have to have any stitches. After the teachers came to fetch him and take him to the nurse for treatment, they called his mother. While Ben sat in the lobby outside the principal's office, waiting for his mother, he panicked and decided to go out of the school and into the street, disappearing down the road. He finally arrived home after hiding in the local park for a few hours.

His parents told Ben that he had to see a counsellor again, and asked him who he preferred to see, as he had seen about four different counsellors, including myself. Ben reached his decision, grudgingly, as he thought his therapy days were over.

His parents were hesitant to medicate him for ADD at the time. They employed a wait-and-see approach because, due to Ben's young age, he was manageable when he became verbally and sometimes physically aggressive. His time-out area was in the small room behind the kitchen. During one of her and her husband's sessions, his mother revealed that they would search the entire house for Ben, only to find him seated on his bean bag in his time-out area, deep breathing and employing the tools he learned in therapy. His father also wanted a time-out area, and so did his mother.

As I remarked before, Ben took to neuron therapy without any opposition. He just accepted it as part of normal life and got on with his counselling program. The approach I used with young Ben was Happy Neuron, Sad Neuron. I got him to draw a few neurons with different emotions on their faces. His neurons were simple figures with faces. They lived in a stadium and played on the soccer field. Ben played soccer and he loved the game, so I used something he could relate to. Two of his neurons were sporty and fast on the field, and another couple were teasers, bullies, picking on the other neurons. Then came a couple of sad and teary neurons, they were always sad and sorrowful, but they were part of the team, so they had to be there. There were also two frightened neurons, who didn't contribute much, but also had to be there. They were frightened and always trying to get out of playing soccer. This was when I asked Ben directly who he was leaving out of the game, as there must be more characters. Ben thought for a moment and said, 'What about the ADD neurons?' I responded by getting him to draw them and wondered how he would illustrate them on paper. But Ben was on it immediately and without giving it much thought. He drew two neurons. They both had no facial expression, only captions above their heads. They had captions attached like in cartoon magazines, showing what the cartoon wanted the reader to understand. In Ben's captions, he had the word 'stupid' on one of them and for the other neuron he had written the word 'angry'. After a moment of awkward silence, I asked him why he wrote those words. He responded that he is stupid because he cannot concentrate and learn, and he is angry because he is a loser. He believed he was incapable of excelling at anything. I prodded him about being good at soccer, and he reluctantly conceded that it was the only thing he might be good at, but he feared that he may also be getting worse at soccer!

Ben's neural network and neurons were all set out on paper, and they were coloured accordingly. His favourite colours depicted the happy, sporty neurons, and the colours he despised represented the sad, frightened and ADD neurons. After familiarizing him with his neuron world and turning them into real characters, I got Ben to oversee all the neurons on paper. He had ten neurons plus the goalkeeper neuron. Ben was now going to be their coach and manager. He was going to be their boss. Instead of them controlling young Ben, Ben was going to manage them. Well, at least learn how to change them to his advantage.

Over the course of subsequent sessions, we concentrated on his neuron soccer team, and I encouraged him to assume the personalities of each of his neurons or players. He was required to portray them and take on their personalities, such as Mr. Frightened neuron or Mr. Sad neuron or Mr. Angry neuron and so on. A few sessions later, I reminded Ben that we should fix those sad and teary neurons because they were not playing the soccer game properly and were putting pressure on the other happy neurons to do all the work; they were making the team lose the game. They were broken. Not working properly. Why were they so depressed, tearful, or angry? And why did two of them exhibit symptoms of ADD? How can we assist them?

You may have noticed that his neurons come in pairs; two angry and two happy and so on. They occur in pairs because sometimes it requires more than one approach to fix the broken neuron. When it comes to children, two is better (and safer) than one. Isolating them from individual neurons may be too overwhelming as we try to repair them. If we have two, for example, and if one does not work, we can then focus our attention on the other one because they are entangled, linked, working as one, anyway. So, if we manage to fix one and not the other, at least there is still a sense of achievement for the child.

Ben's homework was to come up with ways of fixing those broken neurons. We also called them 'broken soccer players'. They were not firing and wiring as they should, or they were not playing soccer as they should.

We began with the so-called simple or less difficult neuron, the melancholy neuron. How could we make this neuron cheerful? How may we assist him? As Ben and I externalized this neuron, transforming it into a real child and a real soccer player, we began debating how we could make this neuron happy once more. It took the entire session, and we were exhausted. At the end of the session, Ben looked at me and said, so how are we going to fix him? Wittingly, I smiled, as I already knew that, from the ideas the two of us just had during our meeting, we were well on the path of 'fixing' this sad soccer player. Innocently, Ben had come up with his own answers during our session. The ideas he put forward were brilliant, and his ideas were what I was going to use to help him fix his broken neurons. We discussed teaching the unhappy neuron how to be happy by engaging in joyous activities or engaging in activities that would make him happy. We also discussed acting techniques, such as pretending to be happy even if he was not happy. *Fake it till you make it!* We also needed to determine whether he was sad for unknown reasons. If so, we were required to resolve them. It was in the best interests of the team for the other neurons to help him recover, as it was in their best interests to win the soccer game. Therefore, this unhappy neuron had to acquire the skills necessary to become a happy neuron. He was required to apply what he had learned. And as the coach and leader, Ben was responsible for ensuring that he acquired these new skills. Ben would hold him accountable and assist him in making these adjustments. And by assisting this despondent neuron, Ben was in fact helping himself.

Next to arrive was Mr. Angry. Consequently, we proceeded until we reached the conclusion of Ben's soccer team neurons. Ben was the private instructor and handler, and the neurons regarded him with great respect. Ben was immediately in charge of a sound team, which are linked to his emotions; neurons firing and wiring together in his brain. By managing his team of ten players and the goalkeeper, he began to manage his own emotions and was able to readily identify them.

Mr. Angry and Mr. Stupid will now be examined. As part of their transition, these two neurons are undergoing a significant makeover, as their coach is unimpressed with their performance. Ben was adamant that they would achieve their objective of becoming Mr. Happy and Mr. Smart. By using visualization and guided imagery techniques, and intention, and pure willpower, Ben was making inner changes, concentrating on his neurons, imagining that he was fixing them from the inside, so these positive changes would be reflected on the outside. By focusing and training his mind to play collaboratively with his neurons, he was preparing himself to be more productive in his outer life, managing his daydreaming and procrastination in the process. By understanding his neurons and how they work on his "inner" soccer field, his fear and doubt became less, and, in turn, his anger subsided. Finally, many of the behaviours of ADD had disappeared altogether, and a new and more spontaneous boy was emerging.

CHAPTER THIRTEEN:
Stephen:
How the Cottage in the Woods Helped Me

No matter how hard they attempt to break the pattern, some individuals cannot escape the prickly side of life. It appears as if they have been plagued or jinxed. It appeared that Stephen was in this faction. He frequently told me that he was the black sheep of the family and that everything he did or attempted ended in failure. In other words, he believed himself to be a complete loser. So, you can imagine how he felt after all his laborious work with me and months of counselling, when something out of the blue plummeted down unexpectedly, proving his point, and reinforcing his incorrect self-perceptions. Even I was taken aback, but we bore no other choice but to stay with his therapy and continue to challenge his negative thinking patterns and challenging behaviours. Still, as they say, the show must go on. His world of neurons was waiting for him, and Stephen was long overdue for a visit.

Stephen was making excellent progress, and he was seriously thinking about studying psychology at university after he graduated from school. His whole outlook changed during his therapy sessions. He was learning so much about himself and human nature in general. He excelled in this area, and I often witnessed his intelligence and insight, but he was quick to shy away from that aspect of himself. He feels more comfortable being silly and/or angry.

Neuron Therapy made him sit up and pay attention. This was something new, uncharted territory, he thought. Stephen wanted to experience everything about psychology, so he eagerly investigated how his brain cells functioned. I recalled when I first talked about neuron therapy and cellular networks, Stephen sat up straight in his chair, watching me with a solemn expression, and exclaimed, "How fascinating!" in a mature and resolute tone. He seemed deep in contemplation, as if this had inspired him. Ironically, during our subsequent neuron therapy sessions, he revealed that as a child, he frequently drew images of different facial expressions. These were simple, circular faces displaying either joyful, sad, or furious expressions. His mother recalled this as well, but she could not recall how he learned about the different facial expressions when he was young. She surmised that she must have discussed this with him or read him a story about various facial expressions.

Stephen needed help getting himself into a relaxed state of mind and body. He needed me to be with him, so we originally started his self-hypnosis and visualization techniques with me present. So, he jumped on my counselling couch and laid back, eyes closed, taking a few deep breaths, getting himself into a relaxed mood. I dimmed the light and ensured no distractions. I was going to be his guide. We began by imagining ourselves in a forest, which I encouraged him to visualize. I was going to enter his psyche alongside him. Initially, he described his forest observations. We needed to concur with what we were observing. I then indicated a wooden cottage in the distance. As we approached it, we expanded upon its description. Thus, we agreed with our environment. There were no other homes nearby. We stood directly in front of the old wooden house. It appeared to have been deserted for decades. No living souls around. Desolate was the surrounding area.

Stephen was lying on my counselling couch with his eyes closed. I could see that he was in the forest, observing the timber home. His facial expression suggested that he was immersed in thought.

I instructed Stephen to wait where he was while I ascended four steps to the house's landing. The ancient, worn-out wooden stairs creaked as I walked up them. As I reached the top, I observed Stephen approaching from behind. I turned and murmured to him to wait. He ignored me while approaching me. Both of us stood at the closed front entrance. I looked at him, and he appeared terrified. I whispered to him once more to remain silent, as there was likely someone inside who was not friendly. We cautiously opened the door. The location was desolate. A musty odour welcomed us. No one was present inside. Nobody was at home. I requested that Stephen describe the interior. There was old and damaged furniture, covered in dust and dirt. Stephen had to memorize the home, both inside and out, because he needed to return frequently to begin working on his neurons.

Stephen could independently access his inner house after a few sessions. He no longer required my presence. Once I was satisfied that he was safe and had familiarized himself with the procedure, I accompanied him once more. This time, I enlisted Stephen as my guide until we reached the old house. He did an excellent job of guiding me to the house, pointing out the small touches he had added to the garden and the veranda to make it more aesthetically appealing. The decorations consisted of quartz-like rocks he discovered in the area and pieces of twisted and peculiar-looking branches that appeared to be ancient and intriguing.

Once indoors, this is where I had to take over because in the far corner was a doorway. The doorway led to another room under the house, the cellar or basement. Stephen was told not to open that door until this day. He opened the door slowly. I stood behind him, watching. As we walked down the stairs, I got Stephen to describe what he was seeing. I added what needed to be added as well. We reached the bottom, nearly ten steps leading steeply down into a dark and mildewed smelling room. Fortunately, a torch was hung near the entrance. When Stephen shone the flashlight around, we observed that the cellar had been emptied. A single worn wooden chair in the corner and a few miscellaneous items on crude shelves affixed to the bulwarks. The bottles and jars of trinkets were dispersed and covered in dust.

I asked Stephen if he could see a mirror anywhere. He said he found a mirror on one of his earlier individual visits; he found it upstairs in one of the rooms, packed behind an old chest of drawers. It was wrapped in an old blanket. "That's it!" I said. Stephen went upstairs and came in with the mirror. It was big and strange. "Pretty cool," Stephen remarked, as he descended the stairs carrying the heavy mirror. It was oblong in form and stood about four feet long and almost three feet across.

Stephen pointed out the intricate engravings around the mirror's frame, and we all agreed that this was an old mirror and that a master craftsman had laboured for months, if not years, to create such an intricate work of art. Stephen wanted to focus briefly on the manufacturer of the mirror, but I encouraged him to move on. The mirror stood upright and reflected his image when he stood directly in front of it after being affixed to a section of the wall of his choosing. This extraordinary mirror appeared to emanate its own energy. Its mere presence alone gave it hypnotic capabilities. It appears the mirror was not only reflecting your image, but also observing you.

Stephen moved a comfortable chair from upstairs to the cellar once he grew accustomed to the strange addition to the downstairs room. I instructed him to position the chair precisely in front of the mirror that never ceases to stare. It appeared to be constantly staring. The instant he sat down, he saw a reflection of himself. But he needed more light downstairs. Upstairs, he discovered four additional torches, which he suspended near the mirror so that he could see what was happening downstairs. As he sat observing his reflection, I encouraged him to visualize and construct his neurons and neural world in the mirror. The mirror was going to analyze his brain cells and then replay them to him in the mirror. He had a rough idea of what his neurons looked like, as I had shown him in earlier sessions, so he knew what to look for and how to bring them to life. After some practice, he told me that he'd started to see a few dim lights flickering in the mirror. When this occurred, his reflection became unclear, as if it were fading away. The more lights that shone, the more his reflection disappeared. Stephen was eventually shown his entire neural network in the mirror. On a vast video screen, he could observe his neurons activating and wiring properly. In the blink of an eye, split seconds of lights lighting up here, there, and everywhere. His interior life appeared bustling and active.

Stephen revealed to me one day that he could manipulate the images reflected in the mirror after a period of practise. If he moved his head forwards to inspect something closer, it was as if the mirror knew what he was thinking and magnified that area. If he imagined seeing something to the left, the mirror would move the image to the left, and so forth. Stephen will soon be able to manipulate the image of his neural world by imagining a location he wishes to investigate. In his imagination, he could also fly over his billions of nerve cells and their active networks at tremendous speed.

After all this fun, Stephen had to get to work. He had to find those dim or broken neurons. Those neurons were responsible for his moods and behaviour, his anxiety, panic, and anger. That's why he is here today. He needs to fix those damaged neurons, and eventually his behaviour.

Stephen is now familiar with his intricate universe of neurons, and he can navigate his neural world in real time, as if he were an expert operating a control panel, as reflected to him by his incredible mirror on the wall. He compared himself to a jet pilot circling his neuron world in search of damaged neurons. He would locate them because he would know where to search. They are typically dim, do not illuminate or shine, and some may even be off and dark. And once he uncovers them, he must send them positive energy to 'will' them to light up again and repair themselves by visualizing the desired outcome. This may require a few visits. Monotony works. He, along with his environment, had altered his neurons over the months or years, moving them off track, so now it was up to him to reset them back to normal. For instance, he had to be specific if he wanted to repair the anxiety neurons. What is the concern? What is the source of the fear? He must visit each of his damaged neurons and encourage them to conquer their fears and liberate themselves from anxieties. Stephen needed to persuade his damaged neurons that a solution was in the works and that everything would work out for the best; that they could trust him. He will safeguard them, allowing them to resume firing and wiring with confidence. Stephen was required to defend them. He was there to assume leadership. He was going to ensure that his thoughts and actions would no longer contaminate his neurons. Additionally, he will visit them frequently to ensure that they are operating properly. Now was the time for Stephen to assume complete responsibility for his neurons and their actions.

On a couple of occasions, Stephen told me that while sitting on the veranda of his imagined cabin in the woods, he would see a man walking through the bushes, seemingly searching for something, before swiftly vanishing into the forest. Stephen found this peculiar. Several times, he observed strange individuals milling about in the bushes without making eye contact with him before vanishing into the brushwood. Stephen called out to them a few times to get their attention, but they acted as if they had not heard him or were unaware of his presence. These strange individuals always appeared to be searching for something, but they never left the forest, staying away from the clear expanse surrounding Stephen's cabin. On one occasion, Stephen decided to approach a man he had spotted through the foliage, but the unidentified man, with a confused expression on his face, swiftly retreated into the forest. When Stephen arrived at his location, he was gone.

I had never heard of this before, as these creations are created by the individual to allow access to their inner and spiritual worlds. I thought that Stephen must have been adding them into his scenery without perhaps knowing that he was doing this, but Stephen was insistent that he had zero to do with it.

I encouraged Stephen to leave them for now and try to concentrate on being in the cottage, rather than sitting on the verandah. He had work to do inside. His mission was to fix his broken neurons that had to do with his worry, apprehension, and wrath. By calming his neurons down and allowing them to glow once more, he had to challenge their faulty thinking patterns and find rational thinking patterns to imprint over the old broken patterns. This would then convert his previous thinking and replace it with fresh thinking. Through repetition and guided imagery, and imagining a better outcome, these individual neurons would change to reflect what Stephen wanted them to produce. And what he wanted them to produce was the removal of fear, overthinking and scary thinking, superseding them with safety, serenity, and contentment.

Things were finally going well for Stephen when he abruptly hit a barrier. He told me that he was familiar with his neuron world and felt comfortable being there, making changes and grooming his neurons to respond to his new way of thinking and being. However, there was an area that he could not go to. At that place, something was blocking him from accessing neurons located there. Stephen asked if it was the Gatekeeper, a powerful neuron or something else that didn't want him to change that bunch of neurons. I hadn't come across this before, and we were stuck. Stephen insisted that he was not creating this himself, bringing about some challenge and excitement into his neural world. I advised him to continue fixing the neurons he could access. Perhaps things would change in the future, and he would be able to return to the location to see if the so-called gatekeeper was gone. However, this was not to be. Stephen was becoming increasingly frustrated because he felt he had lost control of his inner world. But Stephen was determined to fight or challenge that entity in order to reach his damaged neurons and repair them. Therefore, he persisted until he was fatigued. I advised him to take a break because he was becoming disillusioned with this task. He had reached a dead end.

I recall the jolt I suffered during that day with Stephen. It was a crisp autumn afternoon in Sydney when he arrived for his session. Strange how you remember particular and sometimes minor things when you experience a shock. While in Stephen's trance-like state and lying on my couch with his eyes closed, he soon became frustrated again. He exclaimed: "That damn thing is here again! Why is it here?" He mumbled something and I only heard the closing part of his condemnation. "That's it. I am going in. If it wants a fight, it will get a bloody fight!" I reminded him to be careful, that was all I could say. A minute later, a look of sheer horror appeared on Stephen's face. I sat forward in my chair and inquired if he was okay, and why the sudden alteration in his facial expression. He became agitated before blurting out, "I know what it is! Oh no! It's a bloody tumour!"

Surprisingly, I have since come across at least two more people since Stephen's case that have discovered organic abnormalities in their head when performing this work. Sometimes our neurons are not firing and wiring as they should because something organic, physical, is preventing them from working. When this occurs, the broken neurons will become dim or switch off completely, not firing and wiring anymore. Sometimes, your psychological disorders can be organically based.

Stephen was diagnosed with a brain tumour, and the specialist said that they could surgically remove it. Stephen has made a rapid recovery, both physically and emotionally. He told me that he was initially scared to venture inside, go back to his bungalow in the woods and peer into that strange mirror that reflected his microscopic world to him. But he eventually did, and described a vacant lot, like land that has been burnt, around where the tumour used to be. It gave him an eerie feeling. But, as he often says, the show must go on!

And finally, strange how our brain works, those men lurking in Stephen's Forest had disappeared after the operation. Never to be seen again. Were they warning signals, somehow sent to that scene, from the brain or from somewhere else, guiding Stephen to search and look deeper at what was taking place in his head?

CHAPTER FOURTEEN:
Patrick:
How Diving Helped Me

As with most severely depressed people, attending regular counselling consultations is the last thing on their minds. Let alone arriving and sitting with another person who encourages them to show their feelings. Deep down, you already think this is a waste of time. Sometimes it can be all too hard, so early dropouts occur. No shows and cancellations are another problem. Many people who suffer with major depression often tell me that they make their appointments in good faith, but on the day of their appointment, they just can't manage to get out of bed or leave the house, so they end up missing their appointment.

The symptoms of major depression are many and varied, ranging from feelings of hopelessness, extreme sadness, worthlessness, difficulties concentrating, making decisions, feeling guilty for no clear reason, insomnia, sleeping too much, weight gain or loss, fatigue, loss of energy and motivation, psychomotor agitation and recurrent thoughts of self-harm and death. These are the main criteria for major depression. And Patrick ticked most of these boxes. The way he carried his body into my office when I first met with him, suggested some form of depression. His motions were sluggish, and his body and head looked limp as if he had no vitality or interest to hold himself upright. He was disillusioned about his situation and had lost his spark for life. He stated that he was feeling stale, ashamed and did not want anyone to see him. He wanted to go away and have no dealings with anyone or anything. It was like his electromagnetic field had malfunctioned and his liveliness was no longer present.

Patrick's wife accompanied him to a few of his early appointments and told me that she was having trouble keeping him afloat; even encouraging him to groom himself was becoming difficult. During one of these sessions, while Patrick was present, she told me candidly that she did not know how long she could continue doing this. And by "this," she meant how long she could continue to live in this manner due to Patrick's melancholy. She was also concerned that Patrick's persistent despondent behaviour was having a negative effect on their young son. Patrick did not respond to her remark, appearing to be miles removed from his mind.

Patrick had visited numerous mental health professionals over the years, and a variety of medications were evaluated. Initially, some medications were effective, but over time, their efficacy diminished, and new medications were prescribed, and so on. Patrick told me that his two hospitalizations over the past two years for combining alcohol and his medication were not suicide attempts, but rather accidents.

His psychiatric history revealed that he had suffered from depression intermittently for over seven years, but it appeared that his depression had worsened in recent years. His files consistently stated, "no suicidal ideation or self-harm," to my relief. However, my research and observations indicated that his illness was deteriorating and that his wife and son were on the verge of fleeing. I was concerned that if she left now, this man's suicidal thoughts could become a reality.

I encouraged Patrick's wife to attend private sessions with me, so I could help where necessary with coping strategies, and how to better manage her husband's illness. Sadly, she had already been there and practiced that. She told me she had been given so many psychological tools over the years while attending counselling sessions with Patrick. But she was desperate, so she attended, nonetheless.

Patrick avoided counselling and mental health people over the years because of his belief system. He believed strongly that counselling was a waste of time, and not for him. Men did not seek therapy, he told me. Because his problems were becoming worse, and with the insistence of his wife, he finally attended therapy again, but he was ambivalent about the outcome. He told me that some approaches helped him, but after a while, he would revert to his depressed mind-set again. He also stated that he was aware of the importance of staying active and establishing a routine, thus allowing him to divert his attention away from negative thoughts and onto other activities. He told me he had tried everything, including medication, but nothing had helped him. There was also talk of electroconvulsive therapy (ECT) and transcranial magnetic stimulation (TMS), but Patrick was reluctant to consider these approaches. I reminded him that ECT and TMS are usually considered when other forms of therapy do not work.

Patrick complained about the various side effects of medications and was concerned about how long it took for a new drug to work, only to find out that his body was rejecting or not properly absorbing the medicine. He claimed that his depression was still there, and the medication was doing little, if anything, other than making him feel drowsy and tired.

Over the years, he received a combination of cognitive, behavioural, and interpersonal interventions from various treating psychologists, and he attended mindfulness training in an effort to live in the present moment. Relaxation classes and more physically demanding classes, such as Kung Fu and Karate, were also tried without success. His gloomy disposition always made a triumphant return.

Patrick used to become rapidly enraged and confused, arguing with nearly everyone, including his wife. However, he had recently become withdrawn and was no longer interacting with others. Patrick no longer had anything to say or offer. It appeared as though he had almost given up.

Meanwhile, Patrick's situation was made worse by the fact that his wife was spending more time with her parents, with whom she had a solid relationship, especially with her father. Unfortunately for Patrick, the father of his wife had little patience for him and his depression, and the strain Patrick was exerting on his wife rubbed him the wrong way. They don't visit anymore because arguments erupted between Patrick and his father-in-law about not pulling his weight around the house. How could he do this to his wife and child? Thus, Patrick was in the bad books there and had little support from his wife's parents.

The chorus for Patrick's wife to move on grew louder. Many perceived Patrick to be a malingerer. Why was he this way, and how could he treat his wife and child this way? Why was he not improving? People do get depressed, but they recover, and so Patrick felt even more guilty and confused as the whispers persisted. During one of our consultations, he stated, "It's only a matter of time before she leaves me."

I had nothing to lose, just as Patrick did. So, neuron therapy was my next plan of attack. I did observe that he was attentive and responsive to my words, which was a positive sign. He was engaged in our sessions. This was also brought to my attention by his wife. She informed me that Patrick liked me and questioned my confidence in him. She was unable to comprehend why I had faith in Patrick, but she found this encouraging.

When I recall the first time I introduced neuron therapy to Patrick, I chuckle. I can assure you that I did not laugh back then. It was a serious matter, and the atmosphere was so dense that, as the saying goes, one could cut it with a knife. However, I recall Patrick's facial expression when I told him about this revolutionary new treatment. He simply stared at me without expression and did not respond. After a lengthy interval, he exclaimed, "Are you serious!?" I observed that he glanced at his backpack next to his feet and then at my office door, giving me the impression that he was about to leave, and I would never see this man again. Despite this, I encouraged him to attempt it. I reminded him that he had nothing to lose. He agreed there.

First, we had to determine how to get Patrick to connect with his neurons. What technique would he prefer? The wife of Patrick to the rescue! She recalled that prior to Patrick's depression, when they were dating, he was constantly fishing and scuba diving. Patrick adored the ocean, and she was unable to pry him away from it. He relished scuba diving and admiring the underwater scenery. This was ideal; a happy memory that served as a portal into his microscopic neural world.

After two sessions of neuron therapy, Patrick was prepared to embark on his voyage. He shut his eyes and relaxed his body. I persuaded him to imagine himself in a rural location surrounded by majestic trees and mountains. As it was his first time, I planned to accompany him. In the valley is a large body of water, a lake, that flows into the ocean in the distance. The lake is crystal clear and reflects a portion of the enormous, skyward-reaching mountains. It is truly a site to see. Patrick was now required to descend to the lake's shore. A small rowboat was beached on the sand's wet surface. The boat contained scuba diving equipment, including goggles and flippers. These flippers were enormous and, if used correctly, could propel the user forwards at an impressive speed. Patrick told me he was familiar with their use.

Patrick described to me the surrounding area, the boat, oars, and diving equipment, right down to the colour of the flippers.

He told me he refers to them as Fins. Henceforth, I was required to refer to them as Fins. We made our way towards the centre of this body of still water. There were no waves, and the water was calm. At times when clouds obstructed the sun's beams from reaching the water's surface, you could see deep into the depths. Patrick was required to remember the exact same scenery for when he returns, so I encouraged him to describe it for me. I would then remind him later if he left any detail out. If you continually alter the setting or location, it will be difficult to return and believe you are there. For neuron therapy to be effective, you must believe that you are present, in microscopic form, alongside your neurons, so that you can perform your intended tasks. For neuron therapy to be effective, you must communicate directly with your damaged neurons in their environment and using their language. And their vernacular is energy. Your thoughts and focus generate energy. So be mindful of your thoughts and desires when you are in your microscopic world.

Two splashes later, the two of us were now swimming in this magnificent lake. I pondered what pleasures or atrocities lay beneath. I was still adjusting to my large flippers, sorry, fins, and I wondered why they were so enormous. It appears to be for increased propulsion. As a young child, I was thrilled to receive only a snorkel, goggles, and standard-sized flippers. And I was happy. But nowadays, it appears that you must have the most up-to-date equipment, such as gigantic flippers, a color-coordinated wet suit, and swimming goggles with UV protection, not to mention anti-smog and mirrored, to participate in modern water sports. I observed that I was wearing a dark blue wetsuit with sky blue patterns running down the sides. I gestured to Patrick to tell me how he was feeling. He replied with two thumbs up. I imagined he was smiling when he did this, and when I looked over at his face, lying on my couch, with his eyes closed, he had a tiny smile on his lips. Patrick was now one step away from meeting his neurons in person.

We reached a subsurface level that felt appropriate. I made signs requesting Patrick to cease swimming downward. He appeared perplexed and responded in sign language, "Why?" I requested a moment's delay while I surveyed the area. We were sixty feet below the surface and could see roughly the sandy bottom below us. We were positioned near the bay's shallow portion.

Patrick appeared restless and again conveying to me what we were waiting for by making hand gestures. They arrived eventually. From the direction of the deep blue, I pointed to the side of him. As he turned to look at what I was pointing at, they appeared. Hundreds, if not thousands, of golden fish with orange and white spots swam in a dance-like manner towards us. They were swimming as fish do, gracefully close together and in unison. They glistened as their scales captured glimpses of the sunlight that had been filtered to reach our location. Patrick appeared astonished and stared at me with wide-open eyes. I've never seen him with eyes as large as they appeared through his googles. He inquired if these were indeed them. I nodded as I swam away from him while instructing him to stay put. As I retreated, the fish swam around him in a frenzied anticlockwise pattern. Patrick appeared bewitched. As they swam around him, I observed him attempting to delicately touch or stroke them. He was smiling.

As I slowly swam backwards while observing this magnificent scene, I observed hundreds, if not thousands, of these fish swimming ever faster around Patrick. I could no longer perceive his silhouette due to the wall of fish, which seemed to reproduce with each circuit, increasing in number and changing colour from yellow to orange to crimson. After a brief while, I yelled to Patrick to tell them to stop moving so quickly and to slow down. They were travelling too quickly. They were making me disoriented, and I pondered Patrick's position in the chaos. They then slowed down and moved away from him leisurely, no longer swimming in a group or school, but on their own. Some of the fish hovered near Patrick, giving the impression that they liked him, while others swam away, but not too far, giving the impression that they were observing him from a distance. I swam over to Patrick, who was treading water where I had left him prior to the arrival of the fish. Did you see that? he asked, glancing at me. I nodded my head. I instructed him to bid them farewell as we had to get back. Patrick exclaimed incredulously, "Are you joking? We are not leaving now!" After some persuading, Patrick reluctantly accompanied me back to the shore.

This was his first time contacting his neurons, yes, the fish were his neurons. Patrick successfully contacted his neural universe. This was an excellent sign for me. Patrick had embraced neuron therapy.

As the weeks progressed, Patrick was fully immersed in his neural world and no longer required my assistance. He told me that this portion of his therapy was therapeutic and uplifting, and that it allowed him to escape the reality of his situation. He added that he felt at ease when submerged in his private lake with his school of golden and orange-spotted fish. In addition, he noticed that some of his fish were not swimming as quickly as others, that some of them had problems with their posterior fins, and that others appeared discoloured. He was aware that these were his damaged neurons, which he needed to repair. How, then? Initially, he was required to detail his concerns, anxieties, and problems on paper. Each damaged neuron or diseased fish represented one of his problems.

Patrick had no will or motivation to, well, survive. He couldn't be bothered about much at all. He didn't care about himself, nor did he have the energy or interest in caring about others. Guilt seemed to devour him. Life had lost its charm for him.

There was nothing to become enthusiastic about or look forward to or protect. The world would be better off without him, and nobody would care anyway if he was alive or dead. He had no purpose. This is what he often told me during our earlier sessions.

Patrick was temporarily removed from his weighty physical world by Neuron Therapy, which, as he previously stated, was a form of escape for him. Some may label it imagination, but he told me he felt secure and free in that world. However, this was not a fun game to be had, rather, this was work to be done. So, I encouraged him back into the water.

When he was underwater again, he was to target the damaged fish and isolate them, encourage them to heal and persuade them to get better, so they can keep up with the healthy fish. Safety in numbers and all that. These miserable, sick fish were lagging and having difficulty holding up with the group. They had no energy or interest in being interactive. They had no problem being behind the crowd. They held no interest in going with the group and being part of the school. Sadly, they did their own thing, slowly and unhappily, seeming to just exist for the sake of existing. Patrick's mission was to fix them, to give them hope. He had to do whatever it might take to heal them and get them to swim faster and be part of the group. They too had an important role to play. They had a purpose. Their role, no matter how trivial, was important, as working together in the group kept them secure. By acting together as a whole, they would present the impression to would-be predators that they were in fact a big entity, much too large to be eaten.

The more Patrick isolated his sick fish and tenderly stroked their slippery bodies, sending positive messages and healing thoughts into each damaged fish with distinct messages of 'heal' and 'you are getting better,' the more he would eventually bring about the necessary changes. This is referred to as the mind-over-matter phenomenon, in which your thoughts cause internal changes that manifest as new behaviour on the outside. Patrick frequently informed me that his little guys were doing well. One caught his attention and became his favourite. Clearly, this little fish had more than nine lives, as he survived formidable predators and escaped death on numerous occasions. As a result, his skin was torn, and a portion of his small tail fin was absent. He swam with a wobble, slowly, but was always able to keep up with the group. Patrick informed me that this small creature was his good luck charm.

One day Patrick confessed something to me. He asked me if it was okay to do what he was doing about fixing his neurons. I immediately said absolutely not. Apparently, Patrick took some of his ill fish—including his special little guy out of the lake and had them in a rock pool on the shore for safety. He was not going into the lake anymore. He was attempting to heal his fish in the rock pool on the shore instead. Patrick was defeating the whole purpose of neuron therapy. He was supposed to perform this work underwater in his lagoon because this was where his neurons were. They do not work on their own. They will only work when together. Neurons need to be near one another. Later, and after a short debate between us, he blurted out that if he put the fish back, they would be consumed by that beast. Apparently, one day while Patrick was in the water trying to fix his fish, he saw a large menacing fish trying to eat his school of fish. They swam for cover, darting everywhere. This scared him, as the large dark fish looked like a freak, a monster. Patrick said it had sharp big teeth. He said he had his little guy and a few others with him, and if he wasn't there that day, they would have surely been eaten.

Patrick had to get back into the lake and set his protected fish free so they could unite with the group once more. They should learn how to exist and protect themselves. Patrick also had to confront his fears and face his demons. He had no control over what might happen in the lake. He had to be strong and accept whatever came his way. I told him I would go in with him next time. However, this session proved distressing for him, and he postponed his following session. He told me that he was feeling overwhelmed. I assured him that what he was experiencing was normal and part of the procedure.

Patrick's psychiatric history reflected what was taking place with his fish, what was taking place with his neurons. I won't go into that detail here; it is irrelevant and not necessary for me to explain other aspects of his past because it is not needed to explain neuron therapy in this instance. I also want to protect this man's background as it involves many people, and this information may identify him or may cause unnecessary grief.

Strangely, neurons imprint everything that is significant in any way. They will hold on to an image or memory, and it will replay itself over and over when triggered. So, Patrick had to wash that memory away. The fish had to let it go. And to let it go, the fish must be fixed first. And to repair the fish, Patrick should try to replace their damaged fins, bringing out the bandage or putting ointment where there is injury while changing its coding and messages in the process. This is when you can change a faulty or negative message into a more rational one. Then, as your fish heals, it will adapt to the new message or vision you imprinted into it. The result will be a healthy fish (neuron) with a new message, a new encoded message. In other words, your broken neurons will now be repaired, and it will be firing neutral messages as it wires with adjoining neurons. All these changes will occur by simply going into your mind and fixing broken patterns of memories or faulty thinking, and anything else that needs attention. Once deep inside your head, visualize the result you desire. And so, using guided imagery, or creative visualization, or through the power of prayer, or counselling and will power, send your healing energies to create the changes you seek.

As Patrick repairs them one by one, they will begin to light up again and act as they should, and as they develop some hope and motivation and start firing and wiring again, so will Patrick.

Patrick did return to the lake with his small companions and released them to the group. On this occasion, I was with him, and he pointed out the distant demon lurking in the depths. This large predatory fish appeared primordial and dangerous, but it avoided us for the time being. Patrick knew precisely what needed to be done. He looked at me with curiosity and then declared, "I know! I agree!" Patrick's mission was to protect his fish and face off against this deep-sea leviathan. He had to eliminate this gluttonous creature because it had its sights set on his weaker fish, particularly his special little one. Patrick knew that it would only be a matter of time before his little companions were torn to shreds if he didn't kill this monster.

The following day, Patrick waited in the darkness, deep within the murky depths, until he detected movement off in the distance. It was the crooked silhouette of a creature that was approaching his hiding place. He was prepared to strike at the appropriate time. He held a machete, a large cleaver-like weapon, in his hand. Patrick had only one opportunity to complete this task, because if he failed, hesitated, or mistimed it, the monster would instantly remove his head.

Patrick gazed over to where his school of fish was hiding and motioned for them to be still. He positioned himself slowly to confront the approaching beast and observed fur. This odd creature was covered in fur and scales. What is it? Patrick observed that the creature's eyes reflected light and that it appeared to have a snout as it swam closer to where he was hiding, apparently oblivious to the impending danger. As this creature moved closer, Patrick's heart was thumping so hard that it was on the verge of leaping out of his chest. What is this repulsive creature, he wondered to himself. It then transformed as it approached Patrick's location. It was now or never, so he charged forwards with great speed, large blade in hand, and brought the machete down with all his strength, striking the creature in the back of its skull. Then, an ominous silence ensued. The turbulent water returned to its normal, tranquil state. Patrick, still in combat mode, conducted a rapid search of the immediate area. Did I get it? Where was that thing? But nothing. Then, some movement, and as he focused his eyes through the ruby-coloured water, his fish appeared, swimming merrily towards him. His little guy wobbled as he tried keeping up, finally reaching Patrick. The fish embraced him like they usually do; encircling him and brushing up against his wetsuit, then as quickly as they came to him, they swam down to the sandy bottom, gesturing for Patrick to follow them. And there on the bottom, was the carcass of the demon. Dead. The little fish were devouring its bizarre-looking body with delight. As Patrick approached the severed head lying apart from the rest of the carcass, he was surprised to see the head of a dog with a feral appearance. Patrick had slain the black dog that had tormented him for so many years, eating away at his psyche. Further, Patrick had halted the perpetually circling creature that forever terrorized his neurons in the lake of his mind.

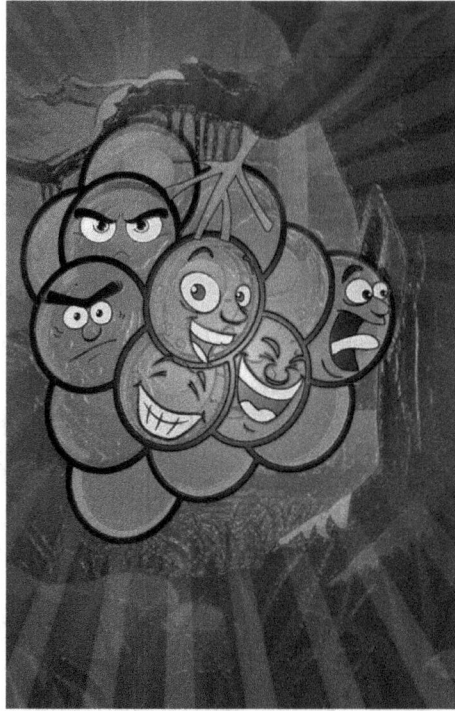

CHAPTER FIFTEEN:
Jacquie:
How a Bunch of Grapes Helped Me

As noted earlier, Jacquie was a well-groomed, professional woman, about to turn forty. She was losing hope of ever finding love and having a family. She disclosed that she was resigning herself to being single and alone for the remainder of her existence. She added that she would share her affection with a few houseplants and a small animal. She had no suitors, and that was that. She was sick of the endless merry-go-round of dating and trying to meet new men. She had concluded that most men were not interested in long-term commitments.

As our sessions continued, Jacquie was more forthcoming with her thoughts and feelings. Either she was meeting all the losers in town, or she was just a bad judge of character, she wasn't sure. I then asked her to elaborate. She told me she had gone out with endless men over the years and most, if not all of them, had some problem that didn't sit nicely with her. She even questioned if her expectations were too high or if she was, in fact, the problem. Nevertheless, she gave up trying to work this out because it was leading nowhere. It wasn't helping her situation.

Jacquie gave me many and varied reasons for men not measuring up to her expectations, including them being self-absorbed, selfish, and controlling. She also added that she had come across some weird guys with undisclosed psychiatric issues. One that was recently liberated from prison, others with violent and pugnacious conduct, two forty-somethings still living with their mother and a few still connected to a former relationship and/or to their children. All these gave the impression that they were not ready for anything long-term. Ironically, a couple of men wanted to borrow large sums of money from her or wanted her to sign into some venture that cost thousands. And last, there were the men who did a runner or disappeared altogether, without giving any explanation to Jacquie.

She also reported that most men she came across tended to fit three categories: narcissist, fickle or passive. From having various interpersonal dysfunctions including self-importance and being unethical, through to the extremely passive and unmotivated. These men were tender and delicate, and lacked decision-making skills, constantly relying on Jacquie to call the shots, to take the lead role, and organize activities and so on.

She asked me why this was so, and why were the men she went out with so unmotivated and passionless? Oddly, she added that the so-called 'normal' men she dated and liked, also had issues, seeming to be confused about what a relationship was all about. Apparently, these men wanted to be single, and only have a relationship when it suited them. Was Jacquie overgeneralizing here?

How then would Jacquie ever find a partner? Where would she discover a man who would fulfil her desires? Was Jacquie herself the problem? One morning during her session, she told me about Mark. He was one of the men she dated briefly in the past. After a dispute over the phone, he informed her that she was crazy and abruptly ended their relationship before hanging up. I asked why that happened and she said that all she was trying to do was to clarify what was going on, as Mark would make arrangements with her and then cancel on the day, telling her that something had come up. This went on for over a month and on this particular day on the phone, Jacquie wanted to address this continuing problem, and this was when he grew furious and ended the relationship with her. I reminded her that on that occasion, she was within her rights to query the relationship and that Mark was being unreasonable, to say the least.

Jacquie found the concepts of visualizations and self-hypnosis distressing, as she was a practical woman. She informed me that she had frequently attempted these techniques after reading about them in magazines and books, believing they were worth a shot. However, she became frustrated while attempting to slow down and visualize aesthetically appealing images. She became impatient and instead decided to tidy the house. Therefore, I had to devise an alternative method for Jacquie to communicate with her neurons.

After speaking about how her brain works, Jacquie appeared confused after learning about the neuroplasticity of her brain and the billions of nerve cells and trillions of synapses found in the brain alone, as well as how cellular learning occurs. She was skeptical and doubtful that she could alter her neural circuitry, but she assured me on multiple occasions that she is open to new experiences and would give it a shot. I guess she was trying to convince herself more than me. Jacquie was also astonished to find out how her neurons make split-second decisions, all on their own, to decide what action to strike next, and how synaptic activity influences behaviour. It's as if there are tiny little brains in each of these cells, Jacquie commented.

I asked her to consider how she could make direct contact with her neurons, as this was the essence of neuron therapy. She stated that she would ponder the matter for a week before returning to her next session with nothing. She was unable to conceive of a way to enter her brain with the intention of repairing her damaged neurons. She told me that she was certain she had a few million damaged neurons that required repair due to her lack of a significant other. The core neuron that is surrounded by other neurons that activate and wire together is the one we must identify. Fixing the primary neuron and its surrounding neurons will have a domino-like effect, causing neurotransmitters to transmit these messages or codes to the others.

One evening as I escorted a client out of my office, I suddenly recalled that Jacquie was a very creative individual. She mentioned her charcoal drawings and expressed her fondness for this form of art. I was now aware of how Jacquie would communicate with her neurons. I proposed my idea to her during our subsequent meeting. It worked flawlessly. Jacquie responded positively and stated that she would immediately begin work.

Jacquie enjoyed gardening and had many potted plants on her veranda and inside her home. She also enjoyed drawing and working with charcoal. These activities were calming and a form of escape for her. She could relate well to them. My suggestion was to use symbolism to make contact with her neurons; the cluster of grapes approach was suggested. She could accomplish this through her artistic abilities, namely her designs. I suggested that she illustrate grape clusters dangling from a grapevine. Simply draw three bunches of grapes dangling from the vine that ran across the page. The bunches of grapes should be drawn sufficiently large so that tiny faces can be drawn on each grape. Individual grapes will be depicted with a smile, a neutral expression, and a sorrowful or ill expression.

The objective was to determine Jacquie's concerns. Then, she had to prioritize them, limiting herself to addressing no more than four issues initially. It would be too complicated to treat her damaged neurons if she had too many problems at once. Therefore, she had to begin with one problem at a time. She could always continue with additional issues in the future.

We identified many problems, including some historical concerns such as an eating disorder when she was in her late teens and early twenties, but she said she had overcome it and that it was no longer an issue for her. I had noticed symptoms of an impulse control disorder when Jacquie became explosive at times, but she reported that these outbursts were rare. I also had just learned that she played poker machines regularly, and soon realized that she was addicted to these slot machines, losing thousands over the last few months alone. She told me that this was one of her few forms of enjoyment. She also talked about concerns with low mood but tried to remain positive as she did not want to get depressed. Admittedly, she told me she felt resentful and angry about her situation and lonely existence but always tried to put on a happy face when with friends. She also added that her father had passed away when she was ten years old and that she did not have a good relationship with her mother.

Jacquie's story was starting to make more sense, but sometimes we need to delve a little deeper into the past to garner all the relevant data. This is important for neuron therapy to be successful. Many issues were present, including anxiety, generalized in nature, and ongoing gambling concerns, which Jacquie insisted was not a problem for her. Abandonment issues and unresolved grief from the past were also present, along with spontaneous verbal outbursts.

How shall we proceed from here? Which of her concerns shall we address first? To make this simpler for Jacquie, we had to consider her current circumstances. What concerns does she have today? She believed that if she had a loving, committed relationship, everything else in her life would fall into place, and she would have a fulfilling existence. I suggested that gambling should be at least second on her list of priorities, if not first, because she was squandering so much money. Jacqueline's top priority was finding a man.

Jacquie arrived for her session with a large art folder. Contained within were drawings of three lots of grapes attached to a vine. We took one of her drawings, as she did three. The drawing was done in charcoal, and it looked lifelike, good enough to eat. Jacquie is a gifted woman.

To help her get settled into neuron therapy I suggested a candle. When she lit the candle, it signified that she was going to work on her neurons. Once neuron therapy was concluded, she would extinguish the candle. The candle would only be lit while she did her inner work. The candle was going to be the association with her neural world. So, Jacquie began by drawing pitiful expressions, which reflected her anxiety and depressed mood. The grapes surrounding the unhappy grapes would have neutral expressions. At the periphery of the group, Jacquie could draw delighted expressions. Next to a sad visage, there would be no happy faces, only neutral ones. According to the hypothesis, the grape with a sad face influences the grapes around it, causing them to lack expression. Happy grapes can be seen further away from the despondent grapes.

Jacquie would begin contacting her neurons through her drawings of the individual fruits once she had completed them. She had a list of issues she needed to address, including anxiety, depression, and impulse control for the time being. However, what prompted her anxiety? What specifically is her concern? What caused her depression? Why was she unable to regulate her impulses? What about her gambling? Her grief? Jacquie believed that all she needed was a loving man and all would be well in her life. Sadly, Jacquie's thought process was flawed in this regard. Before she could discover the ideal man, she had to work on herself. It had absolutely nothing to do with the men out there and everything to do with Jacquie's psychology. Obviously, there are jerks in the world, but there are also decent men searching for genuine love. Was Jacquie just unlucky over all these years?

There is a saying out there that you need to be secure within yourself before you can be secure in a relationship. If two people come together, they should both be whole for the relationship to be enduring. Two halves do not constitute one whole. It just makes a mess. So, was Jacquie looking in all the wrong places? A man was not going to fix Jacquie's anxiety, or depression, or impulsivity or gambling. Was a man magically going to address her past unresolved issues about abandonment, loss, and grief? And finally, is there a man out there that is going to somehow step inside the shoes of her first love all those years ago, and play the role of her fond memory of what she thinks a perfect relationship should be? These and more were unspoken words, emanating from broken neurons, captured and recorded all those years ago, playing these messages now and again for Jacquie's benefit, whether she liked them or not.

Her depression could be a result of unresolved matters from the past (death of her father and the breakdown of her long-term relationship with her first partner) and currently, the loss of money through gambling and loneliness. Jacquie's impulsivity is a form of retaliation for engaging in activities detrimental to her emotional and financial well-being. Repeated occurrences of this behaviour made her situation worse.

Jacquie was required to separate herself from her emotions and begin repairing her individual grapes (neurons). She began with the death of her father. She was going to assist her sorrowful grape drawing in coming to terms with its loss. She had to send encouraging messages and devise practical means for the grape to recover. This grape had been emotionally hemorrhaging for many years, affecting the surrounding grapes. It required Jacquie's input and influence in order to recover. Only Jacquie understood how to heal this grape. With my guidance, she moved through the stages of the bereavement process using this grape. She devoted time honouring her father's memory, bringing closure to the grapes hanging from the vine. She even chose the name Sashi for the grape. When she was a young child, her father affectionately called her by this name.

By working on her grapes in her drawing, she gave them names and brought them to life. During this exercise, inner changes were also occurring in her neural world.

The next damaged neuron, or frowning grape, was her first partner, who left after nearly five years of a happy relationship. Jacquie's heart was shattered then, and it remains broken now. She also needed to bring closure to this memory. She even drew a split heart with a pointing arrow to the sad grape. This grape symbolized her one and only genuine love.

Jacquie took on the therapist's role, and the sad grape was her client. She was going to help that grape get better and move on and start living life again. I helped her with techniques and managing strategies to bring closure to that relationship, presenting her the tools to teach her grape how to let go and trust once more. Jacquie found it less painful to externalize her emotions, hence taking on a counsellor's role, where she was encouraging her broken neurons to heal.

Sometimes in face-to-face counselling sessions, clients have difficulty responding to the techniques or skills taught, however, transferring those methods to your neurons, as noted in this book, seems to work more effectively, rather than absorbing the information personally. In other words, helping 'someone else' seems to be easier than helping oneself. That *someone else* can be your neurons, which may just make therapy more successful, as in Jacquie's case.

Another grape involved stress and being impulsive and highly strung. She drew wavy lines around the grape indicating that it was shaking or shuddering. Its effect was intended to show it being stressed and hyper. An adjoining grape was her worry grape, and it too had some squiggly lines around it. These two were close to each other. Sadly, these grapes are also fake at times. They act passively and pretend to be extra courteous to make people like them. They don't address problems at first because of fears about being rejected, and they don't like confrontation. They then allow issues to persist. They misrepresent themselves as agreeable lambs. They present themselves as something that they are not. After a period of being so accommodating to everyone, being used by others, they eventually become angry, and then a new personality emerges. One moment, the individual is passive, and the next, confrontation and fury erupts. The wolf appears, and there is no sign of the accommodating lamb anymore. And this was Jacquie's life.

Jacquie had to explore why these two grapes in her drawing were like this. Why couldn't they simply be themselves? Why couldn't they just trust? Why the games? These are usually born out of fear. What frightened these neurons so much that they took on these new and conflicted personas? These are the questions Jacquie needed to answer to encourage her neurons to be forthright, confident, and honest. And to be forthright and confident, they had to reclaim their individuality. They needed to understand who they were and what they wanted in life. They should have defined values and objectives. Who are they? Why do they exist? What is their actual function? Jacquie needed to help those neurons come to terms with themselves so they could be strong once more.

As Jacquie continued with neuron therapy, she realized what was going on with her. Separating herself from her emotions and helping her grapes recover was far easier than concentrating on herself and her troubles. By externalizing her emotions through symbolism and drawings, Jacquie was doing great work deep within her own mind, without even realizing the rapid and inner changes taking place in her brain. New neural networks were being organized. Old faulty thinking codes were being replaced by new and rational data, allowing her neurons to fire and wire again, as they should.

Jacquie also realized that she was an insecure person and had many unresolved issues that she thought she never had. The gambling side of things was to do with escapism, trying to get some control and power over her life by feeding a machine with money. But she was going about this all the wrong way. Dating men, without recognizing who she was and what she wanted from them, only made her situation worse. Imprinted on one of her neurons were encoded messages of her first love, and that all men thereafter should live up to his standard no matter how unrealistic that may be. Jacquie subconsciously compared men's qualities to those of her first love.

The other broken neuron had to do with abandonment issues. Her first boyfriend abandoned her, and so did her father when he passed away. Traumatic events such as these can change neurons. Is that why the two neurons changed their roles? Being extra nice and friendly at first, and then shifting to the extreme opposite when their patience runs out? Was this merely a coping mechanism? A defensive strategy?

Did Jacquie have an unrealistic estimation of what men should be like? Had she decided along the way that they were not worth her while? Were they going to abandon her anyway, as significant men in her life do? Was Jacquie sabotaging her relationships without even being cognizant of this? Was she still living in the past, twenty years before, with the same expectations as when she was a lot younger? Were all of these going against her about finding and sustaining a healthy relationship?

When we reviewed her neuron therapy sessions, I inquired about her opinion. She addressed some of the prior concerns. When I summarized my understanding of the situation for her, she became pale. She appeared alarmed when I pointed out the unresolved issues surrounding her father's death, her attachment to the memory of her first partner, and her use of these as a model for all men. Moreover, because she had a secret dread of rejection and abandonment, had she unwittingly sabotaged her relationships and ended them before the men did? She did not want to be abandoned again, so she abandoned herself before they could, without even realizing what she was doing. But her neurons knew.

On occasion, Jacquie manipulated the behaviour of these men to validate her false beliefs about men and their desertion tendencies. Jacquie was clinging to a no-longer existent ideal. She was living in a fantasy world, deceiving herself with flawed and irrational thought processes that were detrimental to her relationships.

Jacquie was oblivious to all of this and could not reconcile the fact that she had been undermining herself the entire time. Perhaps she had dated a few decent men, but due to her anxieties and unrealistic expectations, she had simply walked away from those relationships. She told me, perplexingly, that she lasted longer with so-called inferior men than with quality men, and only now did she realize why she did this.

When Jacquie realized what messages, her damaged neurons were transmitting, she began to cry. As a result of this disclosure, she became extremely emotive at one point, slid off her chair and fell into a heap on the floor, and assumed the foetal position. When she finally stood up, she glanced at her drawings on the desk and, in a fit of rage, attempted to destroy them, blaming her predicament on her drawings of grapes. By performing this action, destroying her drawings of neurons, she would be symbolically destroying her actual neurons in her head as well. Being angry at her neurons would not help the situation, it would only separate her from herself even further. The aim here was for her to work with her neurons and honour them, not hate them.

It took about a week for Jacquie to accept what was happening to her. After that confrontation, I was surprised by how rapidly she adapted and accepted her situation. Jacquie informed me that she had spent the entire weekend drawing, playing music, and absorbing the session in her own unique manner. Her initial inclination was to blame me and her illustrations for her predicament. However, she realized that this was the result of her defective neurons. She also realized that externalizing her emotions, as opposed to locking them up, was advantageous for her. Additionally, concentrating on each grape made it simpler for her to connect with her neurons. She could now use her drawings to enter her brain, make contact with her neuron world, and express her neuron experiences through her art.

CHAPTER SIXTEEN:
Matthew:
How my Old House Helped Me

Matthew was at the end of his road in terms of coping with his condition. Matthew was suffering with post-traumatic stress disorder (PTSD), a term many older people will associate with shell shock. Because of this disorder, and like many other upsets, if left untreated, the individual will try to find their own, and sometimes risky, way to handle their emotions. Numerous individuals use alcohol to contend with distressing or painful memories. Marijuana use and cigarette smoking are two examples. Other substances, both illegal and legally prescribed, are accessible. Overall, these are merely temporary measures that, sadly, do not help the individual recover or return to normalcy in the long run.

Psychological therapy is the preferred treatment for PTSD and numerous other psychiatric disorders. Medicine can also aid in stabilizing emotions and regulating temperament. Matthew had unsuccessfully attempted therapy over the course of his life. He reminded me repeatedly that therapy always seemed to initially benefit him, but that nothing had changed for him afterwards. Fears and night terrors persisted, and he unwillingly proceeded down the path of substance abuse and poor mental health.

Matthew provided me with his previous psychological records, and I observed that he had only attended about ten sessions before dropping out or cancelling them. After approximately four years without support, I observed that he resumed therapy with a new counsellor, before terminating therapy there again. This was Matthew's pattern: he would begin therapy, then abandon it and switch counsellors before moving on. There were extended periods of no support.

I asked him why this was so, and he told me that the therapy sessions were not working for him, and he felt that they were not helpful. I suggested that perhaps he didn't give them the opportunity because he didn't stay around long enough. He responded by asking, 'How long is long enough?' I think back to my grandfather's saying when he couldn't answer my questions when I was a child: 'How long is a piece of string?' He used to say. I don't like that phrase.

Matthew updated me on his symptoms and complained about repeating himself when seeing new therapists, but he reluctantly accepted that this was all part of the process. As was previously indicated, his diagnosis met the criteria for PTSD. After the death of his closest friend when he was sixteen, he continued to have flashbacks, relive the trauma, and feel physically ill. He had difficulty falling asleep, was hypervigilant, easily jolted, and felt guilty. These had diminished over time, but returned in his twenties following the armed robbery where he was assaulted. He continued to relive those experiences; he described hyper-arousal and avoidance symptoms; he became snappy and irritable at the drop of a hat; and he continued to self-medicate with alcohol and narcotics. Self-imposed exile was yet another obstacle that Matthew had to overcome.

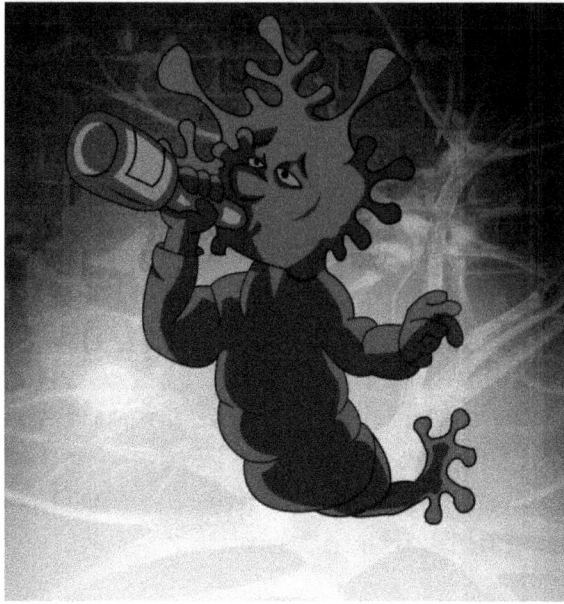

As previously stated, Matthew came to me as a last resort. Both I and he were initially unaware of the nature of his presenting issue. Matthew presented in his first session intoxicated and high. He repeatedly reassured me that he was good to continue therapy. I reminded him that I could not continue the sessions if he continued to show up drunk or high. It was our first significant obstacle. To me, his presenting issue was alcohol and drugs, but I quickly realized that they were a cover for a larger issue, PTSD. What do I address first? I knew one thing for sure, Matthew had to control his alcohol and marijuana use because it was unrealistic for him to attend therapy sessions while intoxicated or high.

Matthew was familiar with supplementary support services such as narcotics and alcoholics anonymous and other support agencies, as well as hospital and university-sponsored training programs to manage addictions and anxiety. I encouraged him to continue, but Matthew did not appear particularly interested. Among others, he was familiarized with Trauma-

Focused Cognitive Behavioural Therapy, Eye Movement Desensitization and Reprocessing (EMDR), mindfulness and relaxation techniques, and exposure-based therapies. Matthew told me he could teach these techniques to students because he had spent years researching them. He was actually a scholar on PTSD and cannabis.

After an initial evaluation, I immediately began neuron therapy with Matthew, as other forms of therapy, some of which had already been mentioned, did not assist him. He was also well-versed in them, so it was pointless returning to them. Matthew gave the impression that nothing from the conventional basket would be useful anyway. He felt defeated and believed that this was his fate, whatever that may have entailed. He longed for something more, something different. He needed hope, and to believe in something.

Since Matthew was already in escape mode with alcohol and drugs, I believed that accessing his neurons through a bunch of grapes would not be effective, so I focused on visualization and self-hypnosis. Matthew was a suitable candidate for self-hypnosis due to his suggestibility. Immediately following a traumatic event, many of my PTSD clients become more suggestible because they are looking for answers and want to normalize their situation. He was also eager to focus on other matters, such as new ideas, so his interest was there.

The objective was for Matthew to meet his neurons, locate the damaged ones, and determine which were the destructive cells, the neurons responsible for replaying the trauma loop and causing him to experience anxiety over and over. His search involved locating traumatized neurons, fearful neurons, addictive neurons, etc. Then he could alter their internal codes and communications. Matthew was required to reprogram his neurons.

As I explained this to Matthew, his enthusiasm grew. This astonished me because he gave off the impression that nothing worked for him. He could be recalcitrant, abruptly abandoning therapy if he felt it was ineffective. Therefore, I found it refreshing that he was finally demonstrating interest in something, as all I had previously heard from him was pessimism about his future.

Matthew wanted me to give him instructions. He wanted to be told what to do. He had no desire to create his own inner neuron universe. He preferred that I describe his cellular environment in detail, and he would embrace it as his own. Occasionally, you will encounter clients like Matthew who are not interested in creating their own virtual world but instead seek instructions and guidance. Therefore, I became Matthew's mentor or, if you prefer, his guardian. I was going to lead him into his mind, and he was going to blindly follow me. Matthew, in desperation, had surrendered his life to me. Nothing else had worked for him in the past, so he would obey my instructions (instead of his own). Neuron Therapy appeared to be his only remaining option.

Matthew's impatience increased. I continued to educate him on how his neurons work, how they send messages, and what those messages indicate if the neuron is not functioning properly. But after a few sessions, he informed me firmly but courteously that he was ready to go. When he arrived for his therapy sessions, he had also complied with my request not to consume alcohol or smoke marijuana. Matthew was arriving enthusiastically for his appointments, and most importantly, he was arriving sober.

After some investigation during his psycho-educational introduction to neuron therapy, I discovered that when Matthew was younger and before the accident on his school excursion, he lived in a large home with his parents and older sister. He had his own spacious room in a two-story residence situated on a large parcel of land adjacent to the foreshore of Sydney Harbour. When he was a child, he frequently played on a small stretch of sand on the beach, just below his backyard, in an inlet along the breathtaking harbour coastline. The residence contained five rooms and an attached guesthouse in the rear of the property. The mansion had a wine cellar in the basement, adjacent to the double garage. Matthew used to play in a tiny room in the attic, which was also a crawl space, located on the second floor. This was his hidden sanctuary. There were vacant storage rooms, an office for his father, and a space for his mother's business. Additionally, there was an old boat shed that contained a small boat and a jet ski. This shed was located close to the water's edge and had a ramp leading into the water.

At the age of 19, Matthew's parents divorced. This came as a shock to him, as he was still battling PTSD three years after the death of his closest friend. His eldest sister had already relocated to England after leaving home. The residence was sold shortly thereafter, and his parents separated. After his parents sold their home, Matthew moved into the apartment they had purchased for him. As his parents did not purchase the apartment outright, he was still paying a portion of the mortgage.

Matthew's childhood home would serve as the entry point to his quantum realm. After drawing diagrams of the house and its layout, like an architect's blueprint, I immediately knew where everything was and how we could navigate from room to room, and so forth. I also learned where he enjoyed being and where he disliked being. Overall, he had fond and affectionate memories of his youth and upbringing in that home.

We began neuron treatment. Matthew always anticipated this day. He had shown me photographs of the house's interior and exterior surroundings, as well as photographs of himself as a young child, so he was familiar with the house approach. I urged him to close his eyes and relax his body by lying down with his eyes closed. I reminded him of the self-hypnosis techniques and emphasized that we had a goal in mind. We were going to go back to when he was a child, around eight or nine years of age. He understood completely.

Following a brief delay, as he initially struggled to visualize himself in his childhood bedroom, he finally found himself there. And I was there, too. He inquired whether we were alone in the room because he sensed the presence of another individual. Normally, there are three of us on these trips, I informed him. He asked who the other person was. I told him that the other individual was his mature self, the one who observes. He explained that it made sense because he was experiencing himself as a child and feeling attached to someone who was observing. I reassured him that the situation was normal and that we needed to move on.

I instructed Matthew to describe the objects in his room, the location of the window, the time of day, for example. As stated previously, he responds to direct questions. He informed me that it is morning because the sun is not by his window in the afternoons, and that he is playing with his football. I requested that he show me every room in the house and explain their purpose. We then went outside where he described the harbour vistas from his backyard. It sounded magnificent. I detected a change in his tone when he mentioned the boat shed, and he quickly suggested we return to the house. I inquired about the wine cellar and attic upon entering. He exclaimed with a murmur, "Oh. Okay," as though he were reluctant to take me there. He very quickly described the wine cellar, telling me that it is boring and has an odd odour, and that he rarely went down there. Even his father disapproved of him playing there, he told me. He has conflicting emotions regarding the attic. He told me that when he was younger, around age six, he enjoyed running and hiding from his parents and sister, but that he was too big to play there now that he was nearly ten years old. He also informed me that changes were occurring within the family. He stated that his family, including his older sibling, were not as happy as they once were.

Matthew was a sports enthusiast and had soccer balls, tennis balls, squash balls, and footballs lying around. His mother was exhausted from putting them away after he kicked or threw them around outside. I explained to him that the balls would eventually become his neurons. He had to take the balls and place them on the floor in his room beneath the window. Matthew was going to familiarize himself with the balls. He would then work on them to change their codes and messages. The balls in excellent condition will represent his healthy neurons, while those that are discoloured or no longer presentable due to age and wear will represent his damaged neurons.

The PTSD and negative thought patterns associated with this disorder were Matthew's top concern. Additionally, he needed to address his excessive consuming of alcohol and daily marijuana use.

When Matthew arrived for his sessions, he would immediately jump onto my couch, close his eyes, and yell, "Ready!" This was his thing. It indicated that he was prepared to reconnect with his neuron world. In addition to being rewarding and surprisingly comforting, he found reminiscing about his childhood memories to be gratifying.

Once back in his mind, I instructed him to begin searching for additional balls in his yard and by the water, as he told me he frequently discovered stray balls, including golf balls, on the small sandy shore. He was instructed to return all the balls to his room and place them on the floor. More balls were preferable than fewer. So, when I entered his room, he described all the balls he had discovered. The room appeared to be overflowing with balls of different shapes and colours. Some appeared to be brand-new and gleaming, whereas others appeared to require a thorough cleaning or to be discarded. However, he was not to discard them. He was required to keep every ball he discovered.

After selecting three dirty balls, he was instructed to wash them in the bathroom. Each ball represented a neuron that had imprinted the trauma and other negative experiences that had occurred since the school incident. Naturally, Matthew was hesitant to revisit that part of his memory, but with my encouragement and while still holding the ball in his mind's eye, he recalled what he remembered from that school excursion. I reminded him that the ball he was holding was comparable to a tape recorder, and that he was required to replay what it had recorded all those years ago. He recalled the sounds, sights, and scents of that day, as well as the chaos of people swarming over him when he first crawled out of the water. As he had never witnessed such behaviour in people before, he found the noises and the frantic movement of the people frightening. Also, he could not comprehend how he felt on that day, as everything seemed surreal. I reminded him to set that ball down and pick up the second one, as the second ball would also contain information about that day's events.

The second ball contained the shocking news that his closest friend had passed away. The image of his friend's body was covered by two wet towels, as Matthew watched on, still seated on the riverbank, with many instructors and students running about in shock. Matthew suddenly ceased speaking while holding the ball. Sadly, after a brief pause, he attempted to continue describing the horrifying events, but his tone abruptly altered, and he became stern. I realized that he had assumed the presence of the Observer, no longer speaking as a child holding a ball but as his mature self-observing the child holding a ball. Matthew had distanced himself from the visceral and agonizing emotions of that day. I signalled for him to take up the third and final ball after encouraging him to switch back to the child. It too was dirty and unappealing. This was the ball of dread and despair. Its message: *nothing is safe anymore and this is going to happen again and again, so you'd better watch out!*

These three balls are his neurons and his house, and the connected rooms and backyard are his neural networks. Matthew had identified his broken neurons and was holding them in his hands when talking to me. He was on the verge of washing them, cleansing them, thereby changing the coding and messages imprinted within the balls. In other words, his aim was to change the level of trauma captured in each of those neurons, so he could manage his symptoms of PTSD more appropriately. Sometimes he had to re-wash those balls to gain a positive result. Put some elbow grease into the repetitive cleaning and programming.

As Matthew lay on my couch in a semi-hypnotic state, I was with him in his mind, sitting in the bathroom with him as he meticulously washed each ball to remove the dirt and negative memories. As he washed the ball, I reminded him that he could replace the unpleasant message or memory with a positive one, or he could attempt to eliminate it entirely. He said he had difficulties altering or removing the memory. Therefore, I persuaded him to continue cleaning the balls for now. Subsequently, he brought out three clean balls. He did a fantastic job. I instructed him to consider what he wanted to write on the balls and what joyful memories he wanted to include. It could be real or fabricated memories from the past. These balls could be used to chronicle anything marvellous and uplifting.

In the meantime, young Matthew continued to manage the assortment of balls in his room and discovered that some were broken and a few required immediate attention, that is, cleaning and reprogramming. Matthew was now at the point where he needed to make those long-overdue, significant changes. In this (reprogrammable) space, he could make any modifications he desired, including imprinting new messages into his neurons, and altering what he wanted them to communicate. Matthew was able to modify his neuron circuitry to generate a new recording that was more favourable than the previous one. He had the ability to make these changes from within his mind, but he seemed hesitant to use it to make the necessary adjustments. Some individuals accept second-best or cautiously coexist with the adversary. Others have chosen to exist in situations that are dysfunctional or detrimental to their well-being. Why change now? Where should I go? No one cares, and I have no significant other. Better the Devil you already know.

Matthew was fortunate in that he did not adopt the victim mentality. He wanted to challenge and alter his neurons and, consequently, his mindset. He had spent too much time with the Devil. But he feared the outcome. What would his future hold? It had become routine and normal for him to lead a solitary, drug-induced existence. Even his darkest terrors and fears were now a part of his existence, so why should he make any adjustments? Is it not simpler for him to remain as he is? After an internal debate with himself, weighing the pros and cons, and confronting his demons, Matthew decided to take the leap and implement the necessary changes. His ambivalence was no more.

He was nine years old when we materialized in his bedroom. His adult self was also observing. Matthew retrieved his coloured markers and proceeded to write on the three balls he had earlier cleaned. On each ball, he inscribed the new message he wanted his neuron to transmit throughout the neural network and beyond. Matthew was reprogramming his neurons, erasing the etched-in image that had been there for so many years. Using various coloured markers, he erased the horrific images from his memory and replaced them with pleasant scenes. He replaced old, dreadful memories with new, fantastical ones by coating over and removing the old ones. It was also essential for him to recreate the same safe and joyful feelings he had as a nine-year-old, as these positive and joyful memories would give him the fortitude to complete the necessary tasks. He had to recall the positive and reassuring feelings and emotions he had as a child to give his adult self the motivation to alter the traumatic memories and end the cellular cycle of repetition. He had to intensify his joy and become euphoric about life. He had to imagine his new memories as if they were real. And as his happy neurons take effect, his new recordings and memories will eventually replace the old ones, sending new communications into his neural network instead of those old, defective, and frightening ones.

Later, it became necessary to address the liquor store robbery. Again, he had to take some balls, this time different balls than before, a total of two damaged balls, and repeat the same procedure as before. He had to clean and repair them. After washing and cleaning the two balls associated with the robbery, Matthew drew new memories on them and altered the robbery's outcome to a more neutral scene. Later, he told me that he changed the scene to show the robbers exiting the vehicle and running past him and his coworker towards the bottle shop's rear exit before the driver of the car fled the scene. In other words, the robbery did not occur in its original form, but a new version of the robbery, devoid of violence and assault, will be reprogrammed into those neurons. The writings and illustrations on the balls were similar to the input of data into a computer system, which programs new information into its memory and other circuits. And when the new information is subsequently requested, it will play the newly programmed messages.

This is one of the processes involved in the modification and reprogramming of neurons. It is an excellent example of repairing damaged neurons, ensuring that they are acting in your best interests and keeping you on course and satisfied with life. Self-hypnosis, visualization exercises, and guided imagery are typically the quickest methods to access and modify your neural world. Nonetheless, individuals vary, so investigation is necessary. Finding the right method is important for neuron therapy to be successful.

I finally asked Matthew why he hesitated about the boat shed when he showed me around his home for the first time. He told me that when he was around seven years old and playing in the boat shed early one morning, a large water rat leapt out at him. This gave him a nasty shock, and since that day he had avoided the boat shed, believing that it was inhabited by large rats. After hearing this, I instructed him to grab one of his clean balls and bring it to the boat shed. I considered confronting his anxieties and possibly erasing that terrifying memory as well. Matthew was eager and made me chuckle when he whispered, "It's not real, it's all in my imagination," assuring himself that the monster rat can no longer hurt him.

The following session, as usual, he jumped on my couch and exclaimed, "Ready!" before entering his mind and reappearing in his bedroom. I was present alongside him. As we headed outside towards the boat shed, he grabbed a tin can just outside the back door, and I asked him what he intended to do with the can. He stopped and declared, "Wow, this is bizarre!" I just remembered the can. This container was used to collect shells by the water. I had forgotten about it. Matthew was amazed by this recollection, as he had forgotten about the pastime he once enjoyed as a child. He collected seashells and kept them in his room for a couple of days because he enjoyed the smell of them. Once the scent had diminished, he would gather more.

He then told me about Isabella, a female who lived across the street. She was the same age as him and they frequently gathered shells together. This was another memory he had just remembered. "How bizarre!" he remarked. Where are all these memories coming from?

Matthew appeared comfortable as he rested with his eyes closed on my couch while guiding me through his thoughts. I was able to visualize what he was describing. As we approached the boat shed with a couple of balls in his hands, he hesitatingly laughed nervously and then cautiously laughed again. "This is only a memory, and I am still terrified," he said, chuckling to himself once more. I asked him to describe what he observed as he opened the creaking door. "It is dark," he informed me. It smells like a boat shed, a combination of gasoline, ocean, and damp wood. The boat is covered with a hefty canvas, while the Jet Ski is partially covered. "Where did the rodent leap from?" I queried. He pointed to the rear corner of the shed. "I was over there collecting shells when a large rat ran along the side of the wall towards the water, directly towards me as I bent over to collect the shells." It was fast and hopped or leapt approximately two feet in the air, causing me to scream.

After lingering in the boat shed with no rats in sight, we walked back to the residence. He spoke once more about Isabella, the girl from across the road. Clearly, she heard him scream, as she was on the shore that day collecting beautiful seashells herself. Matthew was humiliated when she giggled at him as he ran out of the shed carrying an empty can. His shells remained in the boat shed. Isabella was the one who entered the shed to retrieve his seashells. "I can't believe I'm remembering this," he said with a previously unseen expression on his face.

Throughout subsequent sessions, I asked him how he was doing, and he reported that he was enjoying the visualization exercises and recalling many happy memories. He remembered his dreams about the future, including how he would marry Isabella, reside on the beach, and be surrounded by seashells. He had forgotten his fondness for seashells until just now. I observed a significant shift in Matthew's mood as he provided me with an update. What is your drinking and marijuana smoking situation? I questioned, dampening his enthusiasm for a moment. "I've cut back," he assured me. He told me that whenever he felt the urge to drink or smoke, especially in the evenings, he would go within his mind and reflect on happy memories from his past. He would return to his childhood home promptly, hoping to catch a glimpse of Isabella and see if she was on the beach, as she frequently was after school and on weekends. Matthew was successfully managing his alcohol consumption, with up to three and four days without any drinking or smoking. It was a monumental achievement for him.

Matthew was continually changing. He was looking more peaceful and content and even began making jokes. He did not make jokes before. But now he was making jokes. One day, from out of the blue, he asked me if I wanted to go with him to check out the old house. He wanted to see if it was still in original condition (or in fact still there!) and if visiting the little beach behind the house would conjure up even more memories for him. I was busy, so he went alone. I wondered if he was secretly looking for Isabella.

Matthew still had a way to go in terms of managing his mental health, but for the first time, according to Matthew himself, he declared that he was feeling hopeful and joyful. He couldn't believe he had reduced his alcohol consumption to twice per week and his cannabis consumption to roughly once every two weeks and diminishing. He was now looking for a new interest to focus on, finding a substitute for his drinking and smoking. He thought about seashells and what he could do with them to make money.

CHAPTER SEVENTEEN:
Cassandra:
How Two Fat Fairies Helped Me!

Cassandra continued her struggle with her weight. This was her life: she would eat healthily for a brief time and feel proud of herself, then binge eat when stressed, consuming excessive amounts of anything she could get her hands on. Cassandra desperately needed assistance with weight management, so she turned to the gym, weight loss consultants, and others for assistance. As a last resort, she sought counselling.

When I first met Cassandra, she presented herself in a bubbly manner and was quite talkative, occasionally losing her train of thought and then laughing about it. She gave the impression that all was well in her life, requiring guidance only with weight management. She inquired about hypnosis because she had read about individuals losing weight through hypnosis. I told her that it may be effective, but I would also recommend self-hypnosis.

Cassandra informed me of her daily schedule and nutrition. I found nothing remarkable or concerning about it. In what she told me, she was eating like a bird. I pondered why she was struggling with her weight and why her final weight was 96 kilograms. She was slightly taller than 5 feet 2 inches. Afterwards, I discovered that eating like a bird was limited to the previous few days. Cassandra neglected to mention the episodes of excessive binge eating.

During our first few sessions, I observed a cheerful person on the surface, but a melancholy and lonely woman underneath. I was able to see it in her gaze. Her face would appear to be beaming, but her eyes told me otherwise. She agreed with my observations after I pointed them out. Then tears suddenly rolled down her cheekbones as she told me more of her history and story. I also inquired as to whether she was aware of the connection between overeating and her emotions. She didn't know about this. She asked me to clarify my meaning. When agitated, anxious, or depressed, people's behaviour can fluctuate, and they may do things that are not considered rational. In Cassandra's case, this included excessive eating, binge drinking, overspending, gambling, becoming aggressive or hostile, and so on. She asked me if it was like having an addiction or obsession. "Kind of," I replied, "but there is a distinction. Obsession is more about ritualistic routines, doing things the same way or at the same time, whereas addiction is more about satisfaction, doing something to get fulfilled, such as a physical brain rush."

"It sounds like I am addicted to eating?" she commented, smiling lightly. 'Even so, you can also be obsessed with food, just to complicate things for you', I said. She laughed and agreed with me.

Cassandra did as much research as she could on neuroplasticity and learned as much as she could from what I had taught her about this topic, so focusing on the theory portion of neuron therapy was not particularly useful. Like most individuals, Cassandra wanted results. She had little interest in the philosophy underlying neuroscience and the proposed treatments involved. She only wanted outcomes, a fast and simple method for managing her emotions so she could control her food intake. So, our work began. The initial step was to create a weekly schedule that included a realistic exercise regimen, dietary intake, and food preparations. She was to keep the plan simple. Cassandra had previously navigated this path, so she knew what to do and what was expected of her. She told me that although the program worked in principle, putting the plan into action proved difficult. What happens if I'm alone at night and have a sudden craving for food? Food makes me feel better and creates a feeling of calmness. Cassandra described an excellent example of comfort eating.

Second, Cassandra was required to alter her dietary habits and daily routine. She needed to be aware of her emotions and how they affected her moods. She would have to maintain a log of her emotions, including her stress levels and anger. She was also required to monitor her emotions of guilt, anger, sadness, and fear. When possible, I encouraged her to consume actual food rather than junk or processed food. We considered reducing her portion sizes and eliminating food groups that were considered unhealthy and fattening. Additionally, we ruled out dietary intolerances and allergic reactions. Cassandra used a small plate for all her meals to control her portion sizes.

Cassandra's enemy was physical activity and water. She informed me that she loathed exercise and drinking water. In addition, we examined her social networks and ways that she could increase her participation in outdoor and recreational activities.

When I first introduced Cassandra to neuron therapy, her eyes lighted up. She adored the mysterious nature of things and was eager to learn more. She could not contain her enthusiasm when I explained how neuron therapy works, confirming that I was on the correct track with her, as she finds this topic intriguing. She admitted that she was interested in astrology and followed her star sign every day; that she frequently contacts psychics and was even consulting a spiritual healer to help her lose weight. She joyfully informed me that she has faith in the supernatural world and that life is comprised of more than just physical matter. I was confident she would be a good candidate for this form of therapy due to her open mind.

I elaborated on how neurons and neural networks in the brain can alter their connections and performance in response to the individual's circumstances. If incoming information is negative and internal thought processes are dysfunctional, neurons will alter brain chemistry to reflect this reality, thereby producing instructions for this reality to manifest physically. In other words, if you believe you are a failure or a bad person, your neurons will make these beliefs true, and it will eventually become your belief system. However, if positive feedback is received, believed, and imprinted into brain cells, then brain cells will communicate that information, thereby producing positive and upbeat messages and physically manifesting them. You are the sum of your neurons. Similarly, your neurons shape your brain and contribute to your identity.

In Cassandra's situation, a great deal was going on for her. She struggled with unresolved familial issues, loneliness and isolation, issues with her diet and weight, and confusion regarding her identity and future plans. In addition, she was an exceptionally intelligent woman who conducted extensive research on her condition in terms of mental health, diet and nutrition, and medication. She was also against all types of medication. She spoke negatively about the pharmaceutical industry's desire to medicate everyone in exchange for billions of dollars. Once she learned about neuroplasticity, she continued her investigation to find out how this new science could improve her life. I was delightfully surprised when she responded with remarks such as, "Did you know that positive psychology can help improve brain structure? Also, did you know that some sections of your brain will shrink or become smaller if they are not used frequently, and grow larger if they are used regularly? Wow! Why isn't this taught in schools and universities?" Cassandra was opinionated, and neuroscience was becoming her new focus. "And those mirror neurons, how strange!" Hence, the origin of the phrase: "like-minded individuals attract one another." "It is all due to mirror neurons!" Confused about what she wants to study at university, I think, just maybe, Cassandra had found her calling.

If you're unfamiliar with the term, a brief explanation of mirror neurons follows. Mirror Neurons enable us to comprehend ourselves by observing others. When we 'mirror' another person, we demonstrate interest in them by reflecting agreeable emotions and behaviours to blend in and be accepted. It is also essential for learning, which involves imitating others to comprehend their intentions and mental states behind particular actions.

During our ensuing sessions, Cassandra was eager to inform me of the latest developments in neuroscience and how this field is transforming the world. I inquired as to where she obtained her information. She swiftly responded, "From Ms. Google." Before I was able to clarify the prefix preceding the search engine, she smiled and stated, "Only a woman could hold all that information." Interestingly, she continued, "If the neurotransmitters are linked to your emotional and behavioural traits or personality, regardless of whether they are positive or negative, is it possible to change them if they are holding you back or causing you pain?" I knew the answer, but I was curious as to how she would respond. I asked her opinion on the matter. Cassandra informed me that her research and readings had led her to the conclusion that the brain is resilient and can rewire or repair damaged brain cells through repetitive thought processes and sheer tenacity. She was on the correct path, which made my job easier.

Cassandra wanted to work on her weight as her primary objective. She yearned to cleanse her mind, eliminate her late-night binges, and reduce her food intake by fifty percent. We discussed realism and the possibility that her expectations may not match reality. Nonetheless, this was Cassandra's goal. She needed a makeover. She wanted to reprogram her brain.

Part of our counselling and therapy often involved shifting attention and interest away from food and finding substitutes or other means to occupy her mind and calm her food and hunger drives. She told me during one of her sessions that she can picture her neurons going berserk because she was depriving them of food. Out of curiosity, I asked her to describe her neurons. She told me that they are all different, and some were obese, while others were full of anger and hatred.

Neuron Therapy facilitates many changes in various brain regions. Particular parts of the brain are impacted by negative thinking that is reinforced by poor behaviour, causing a disruption in brain circuitry, and your neurons will reflect this. In turn, your emotions and feelings may be compromised, which may manifest as moodiness, anxiety, anger, and so forth. There is now evidence that creating a new reality through positive reinforcements, such as visualization and self-hypnosis, physical and outdoor exercise, and feeling cherished and valued, can make a person happier. Laughing and being content with life are also essential. Finally, gratitude is crucial and can contribute to the creation and maintenance of a positive neural network. And when your neurons are properly wired and working correctly, homoeostasis will occur between the body's biological processes, including the energy component of your being and the electromagnetic field that surrounds every part of your body.

With all the virtual and psychological tools in place, the next step was to introduce Cassandra's neurons to her. According to her weekly planner, she would take a steamy bath every weeknight to unwind. This was designed to prevent her from cooking in the evening. The objective was to calm her entire being. This was also a component of her weight loss regime, which included psychologically regulating her stress levels and making contact with her neuron world.

Since Cassandra favoured Metaphysical and Quantum Therapy (MQT) so much, we opted for this method. Before entering an altered state of mind, she planned to relax her body in a hot bath with candles burning and gentle relaxing music playing in the background. The warm, fragrant water would help place her in the proper frame of mind. MQT is essentially a technique in which you imagine yourself in a different location or dimension. It is not a form of meditation in which one relaxes and finds serenity, but rather a form of self-hypnosis in which one has a particular goal in mind. You have a role with an intended outcome. In other terms, you are actively reprogramming information in your quantum world while participating in your mind's eye.

Cassandra informed me of her MQT results during her sessions. Initially, we attempted the exercise in my office, as I do with all my other clients, but Cassandra preferred to perform the procedure in the privacy of her own home and bath. She told me that, over the years, whenever she took a bath, she would unwind and enjoy herself by fantasizing about a variety of fun things for approximately an hour.

Cassandra reported that she was initially unsure of what scene to compose, but after letting her mind wander, she found herself in a magical forest with some strange looking but innocuous small furry creatures. Everyone there was pleasant and made Cassandra feel welcome. There were also minuscule flying creatures, so Cassandra had to use her imagination to make herself small as well. She observed, in her microscopic form, that these flying creatures were tiny fairies. Upon closer examination, their tiny wings were translucent, like those of a dragonfly. Their tiny bodies were concealed by a maroon garment that glistened momentarily. They had tiny hands and feet. Their eyes were deep-set and large in their small heads. When they flew close to Cassandra, she could hear their wings flapping. They lingered in the branches and had nests made of leaves, whereas other fairies lived in holes dug into the bark of the ancient, majestic trees.

This newly created kingdom was Cassandra's quantum world. By entering and reducing her physical size to match the little fairies' size and to enjoy their tiny world, she had to become minuscule. And to gain entry there, she had to go through her bath.

Cassandra was a fan of fantasy-themed computer games and films, and she told me with a broad grin that as an adolescent, she had mastered many of the available multiplayer online games. She frequently chose to play bizarre characters, preferring to be the queen warrior or evil princess, saving, or destroying innocents from the hideous creatures that lurked in the game's virtual domains.

She informed me that her narrative was already in motion and that she was in contact with her neurons in her magical kingdom. She had already discovered several broken ones. She also told me that the happy neurons (fairies) were flying aloft and appeared healthy as they darted from flower to flower in the beautiful meadow. She had also observed a pair of fairies moving slowly through the land's vegetation, no longer flying, and giving the impression that they were bearing the world on their tiny shoulders. Their wings appeared defeated and pitiful. She informed me with reluctance that they were the two obese fairies. Their delicate little wings were incapable of lifting their enlarged bodies off the ground, so they were forced to walk everywhere. How they yearned to soar once more!

Her description of her newly created neural universe sounded familiar, and it is likely that many young girls will identify with her sentiments. Cassandra appeared content as she created an inner universe filled with exquisite landscapes and exotic creatures. I also reminded her to stick to the plan for identifying what she wanted to work with, how the characters would represent the messages she wanted to alter or fix, and the roles of the other creatures in her microcosm. This is a crucial issue. Creating or visualizing too many characters and projecting a complicated setting would not only lead to confusion but would also make it extremely difficult to retrace your steps when returning. I had to remind Cassandra to maintain a simple inner universe. Do not construct characters or settings if they will not contribute to the management of one's mental health. Keep things simple.

Cassandra remarked that she had created all these enemies beyond the gates of her inner world and realized that she did not understand their purpose. She finally pruned her interior game, resulting in a modest village. A creature that abducted and enslaved young fairies resided in the gloomy, hostile forest beyond the horizon. Cassandra ruled over her domain and was also a ferocious warrior. No one dared access her kingdom without an invitation, much less kidnap or harm her small flying subjects.

Cassandra urgently desired weight loss. In addition, unresolved issues from her past had caused a negative recording in her brain, a broken synaptic loop that prevented her from being free and joyful. Several of her neurons were not activating and wiring properly. She had a pattern of preventing her own happiness and resiliency. She engaged in negative self-talk and frequently experienced unjustified dread, preferring to be alone and in what she perceived as a safe environment. Her idea of a secure space was to not trust anyone. Therefore, being alone at home with food was all that she required. It was convenient. It was dependable. No confusing emotions or disappointments. In fact, she had plenty of experience with that in the past.

Remember, initially, neuron therapy involves keeping things simple. Concentrate on a single task at a time. Cassandra agreed to focus on her weight problem for the time being, so she had to concentrate on the two neurons that had become too heavy to fly. If these neurons weren't sleeping or unwinding in their leafy hammocks, they were leisurely foraging for food. They relished ice cream, all types of sweet pastries, and savory meat pies with sauce. These were Cassandra's preferred late-night delicacies.

To communicate with her neurons, fairies, Cassandra was required to meet them as their Queen. She needed to impart to them a sense of purpose and value for them to feel motivated to be productive and effect change. This was the mission of Cassandra. She accepted the responsibility of caring for them and encouraging them to make positive adjustments in their lives as their queen.

Cassandra has since learned that one of the obese fairies recently suffered a loss and was in mourning. The other heavy fairy felt unloved by the world and was lonely. These neurons had resigned themselves to their fate and were patiently waiting for circumstances to alter their destinies and take them away. They were in a state of limbo and had little to anticipate. They were merely present. As a result, food alleviated their suffering, erasing their feelings of worthlessness and despondency.

At this point in her therapy, Cassandra was reacting negatively to the influx of information and could not believe how her neurons mirrored her life. It was as if they had recorded every detail of her past and were now selectively playing back the most distressing portions. Through her emotions and actions, a portion of her vast neural network was manifesting its distressing messages and defective signals. Why? The answer is quite straightforward. Whatever enters must also exit. In other terms, our neurons store all information, positive and negative.

These recordings are the result of internal factors such as ruminating on negative thought patterns, hypocrisy towards oneself or others, and excessive concern over trivial matters. Environmental factors, such as observing or experiencing a traumatic event or being subjected to prolonged stress, may also influence neurons. Then, if they are not processed properly and assimilated into the brain, they will be played back to you at unexpected times, like a tape recording.

If your neurons are broken, as suggested in this book, you will need to reprogram and alter the defective signals they emit. Occasionally, the entire neural network may be affected by past traumas and negative memories. In Cassandra's case, issues from her past relating to abandonment as well as her belief that she was in some way defective, a monstrosity, and not desired by anyone needed to be addressed. She once told me that the word 'broken' is appropriate because this is how she perceived herself for most of her life.

Cassandra had to convince her two fairies to lose weight so that they could once again take flight. In addition to helping them reduce weight, she had to assist them in burying the past. They needed to reinvent themselves and flourish. This chapter in their life had reached its conclusion. They had to begin a new chapter, narrative, or objective. In other words, they were required to reinvent themselves for a new period in their lives. Living between chapters resembled a state of being in limbo. Living in the past with chapters already lived was regressing, which typically results in grief and sorrow. Cassandra (and her neurons) had only one option for moving forwards, and that was to begin writing the next chapter in her life story.

Cassandra possesses a profound spirit and a fantastic imagination. She has always felt that her weight has held her back from engaging in so many inspiring and creative activities. Her apartment was filled with various forms of fantasy-related content, including novels, magazines, DVDs, toy models, and more. She was also an avid online gamer who delighted in battling and defeating opponents from all over the globe. Cassandra's next step was to not only penetrate her neuron world, but also to enter the neuron itself. When I informed Cassandra that this would be difficult, she responded that she was ready and waiting. Definitely the response I wanted.

Cassandra was adept at fighting in the virtual world, and now she would enter her own cells to fight against faulty programs that had been placed there in the past. She intended to correct the detrimental internal messages.

Cassandra was a diligent student who took notes on her dog-eared notepad after she was instructed on what to do. She drew pictures alongside her writings to illustrate what I had instructed. I answered her queries when she raised them. She responded to my questions, demonstrating that she comprehended what was required of her. Cassandra was now prepared.

Cassandra always told me that her brain appeared to be sharper when submerged in water in her bathtub; creative ideas came to her there. Also, she could solve difficult problems when sunk in warm water. So, she would use her bath to enter her microscopic universe through the power of her imagination.

She greeted her two obese fairies when she came across them while they were strolling in her newly created land. They were transporting food back to their home in the hollow of an old tree. Cassandra invited herself to join them as they prepared their afternoon meal while she visualized the scene in her bath. There was just enough space for the three of them to sit comfortably inside their minuscule, carved-out dwelling, with the door slightly ajar to allow natural light to enter. One of the obese fairies ignited candles on the opposite side of the room to provide illumination. Cassandra observed these two tiny beings as they prepared a snack. Strangely, they prepared their meals the same way Cassandra did, even eating some of the ingredients as they prepared them. In addition, they drank soft drinks to stay hydrated while preparing the dishes. Pastries, surprisingly Cassandra's favourite, were on the menu. Cassandra appeared to be observing miniature representations of herself in action. This made her feel uneasy because she could see what they were doing and how food-obsessed they seemed to be. It appeared that every waking instant was devoted to deciding what to consume next. While they were still preparing their late supper, these neurons communicated with one another about what they would have for dinner. These neurons, fairies in Cassandra's imagination, were stuffing their faces with snacks and carbonated beverages while baking apple-cinnamon pastries. Additionally, they made pies with meat and sauces. The plan was to start with the meat pies and conclude with the apple pastries. The ice cream was also prepared, but the question was, which flavour? This was quite a conundrum. Vanilla and strawberry were equally delectable, as were chocolate and rum and raisin.

Cassandra had shrunk herself to match the size of her neurons in her exquisite land, where she replaced her neurons with living fairies going about their day, firing, wiring, and transmitting messages, as they normally do. However, Cassandra was now required to reduce herself even further. She had to shrink herself below the size of her fairies. In this case, the objective was for her to enter her fairies, or brain cells. The goal was to alter the message within the neuron itself, prior to its transmission into the network.

Cassandra had to will the fairies to sleep after they had relaxed while awaiting the pies. Remember that Cassandra controls the inhabitants of her inner world. Cassandra planned to imagine herself inside one of the sleeping fairies once they had fallen asleep. She planned to shrink herself even further. And then, and so quickly, she realized she was in a large circular chamber. She was within the neuron itself. It reminded her of a large water reservoir supported by four tall beams, a scene she frequently witnessed in American rural-set films. Inside, it sounded hollow. In this spherical chamber, there was a steel ramp leading downwards from near the ceiling. It appeared that workers utilized this ramp to access the walls and make any necessary repairs from within. It was a platform upon which they could stroll. As it was a steep descent to the bottom, the workers were protected by a steel fence that reached their waists. There was a round opening at the bottom through which water or other liquids could escape or drain. This opening was obstructed by a trapdoor. Using the trapdoor, it could be controlled to keep whatever in or let whatever out as needed.

Attached to the wall and spiraling downwards, these circular footpaths were on various levels of this enormous dome-like structure with a round-like shape. There was one on top, approximately ten feet down from the round ceiling's apex, another one midway down the room, and a third one near the bottom. Therefore, whoever had to perform work there could move from the top down, ensuring that all walls were accessible from those platforms.

Cassandra was atop the highest platform. The interior appeared terrifying and bizarre. As her eyes adjusted to the dim light, she was able to see writings scattered throughout this circular chamber. As she looked downward, she noticed that there were writings on the walls everywhere, even near the drain opening. A portion of it resembled graffiti. There were scratches and torn sections of old paint dangling from the ramparts, along with messages that appeared to be deteriorating over time. In addition, there were new and lucid writings. Cassandra was astounded when she recognized the words. The inner walls of her neuron, the interior of this circular chamber, were covered with writings and slogans that conveyed a clear message of humiliation and shame. Hundreds, if not thousands of messages: "I am overweight and unattractive!" And "I am worthless!" And numerous other mocking phrases that were upsetting to observe. It was as if a vandal or a nefarious thief had broken into your home and scrawled those horrendous messages on your walls, implying that you are worthless and have no purpose in life. Also, "I am a freak!" and "Everyone hates me!" and "No one will ever love me!"

But then, as if by instinct, Cassandra knew she had to brace herself by bending over and gripping the railing, as the trapdoor below suddenly opened and a whirlwind-like suction sucked the air down, pulling anything that was not secured through the trapdoor below. Cassandra held on for dear life as the downward pressure nearly tore her hair from her scalp. She held on tightly because if she let go, she would be instantly pulled down. Just as quickly as the trapdoor opened, it slammed shut with a deafening bang. After the trapdoor slammed close, everything stopped, and calm was restored. Cassandra stood up and observed that the writing on the walls had been removed. Most of them were gone, perhaps sucked out of the trapdoor below. As she attempted to comprehend what had just happened, to her astonishment, the writings reappeared, as if by magic, with the same degrading and unsettling messages as before.

What was happening here were simply neurons doing their job, firing their messages into the network, and conveying what was written on the inside to the outside as a reality. This neuron was damaged because it transmitted erroneous signals. Cassandra was tasked with repainting the entire wall and rewriting messages that were beneficial to her welfare. She was able to use the path that spiraled downward from top to bottom. She could use the platform to access these writings and demeaning messages. She had to paint over them quickly, as that trapdoor opens often.

Cassandra painted over the embarrassing and excruciating writings and memories with a paint roller, holding on for dear life when the trapdoor suddenly opened and sucked her new paint off the walls, revealing the writings and memories underneath. Once Cassandra realized that the suction from the opened trapdoor made it more difficult to remove the dried paint from the walls, she painted with greater fervour and speed. When she was certain that most of the paint was no longer coming off, she moved on to the next phase. She now had to paint new messages and images on her newly created canvas using a paintbrush. These writings could be neutral or positive in nature, anything she believed would enhance her mental and physical health. Cassandra wrote, "I do not need food to survive; I will survive without excessive eating." Other anxieties and memories she replaced with happier ones or removed entirely, replacing them with fantasy-based stories that portrayed her as the hero or the wise woman.

Some sections of her freshly painted wall were already showing symptoms of deterioration due to the notorious trapdoor's wear and tear. Again, she was required to act swiftly and redo them until the paint dried and the new message became permanent. This new message is transmitted to the brain and all its connections, including her central nervous system and electromagnetic field, when the infamous trapdoor opens. Even if they are momentarily pulled off the walls by that trapdoor, her new writings and memories will now reappear, fairy-like, because Cassandra changed the coding, the erroneous message within her neuron. Therefore, her new message will now be transmitted throughout her neural system and synapses, as well as beyond. As programmed by the network's owner, the transmission will eventually propagate throughout the vast neural network. In other words, Cassandra had now Neuro-hacked her brain to produce the outcomes she wanted.

A brief quantum perspective on Neuro-hacking and Neuro-engineering. Simply put, it involves rewiring your brain. These terms are used to describe neural networks and how they are susceptible to external and internal hacking. The objective here is to determine if you are being Neuro-hacked by external assailants or if they have already programmed you! Have you been indoctrinated or programmed in a manner that is detrimental to your well-being as a whole? Or have you, through years of negative thinking, Neuro-hacked your own brain to produce the outcome you now, see?

Neural networks are magnificent brain cells that can be programmed and arranged to reflect their input. These could be traumatic or blissful experiences; either way, they will be assimilated and stored in our neurons and other brain cells for later replay. Neuro-hacking is the act of hacking into one's own brain to repair oneself or remove potentially harmful recordings that other hackers (or oneself) may have placed there.

Cassandra's final mission while inside the body of her fairy, the round hollow-sounding chamber, was to leave messages on the three landings. She was required to establish new objectives and a clear path. Her goals should be reasonable and in line with what she hopes to accomplish. In addition, Cassandra had to reinvent herself by appreciating her natural talents, enhancing her assertiveness, and designing a future that reflects her personal values and passions. She required self-discipline to accomplish her goals. Her objective was to lose weight and keep it off. So, a component of this goal was to include a strategy of how she was going to implement her plan.

Now that some of her neurons have been repaired through Neuro-engineering, Cassandra would find this task somewhat simpler to complete. Improving yourself and making necessary changes is difficult with a healthy brain, and it is even more challenging if your brain is sabotaging you along the way. Changing the coding and messages within the damaged neurons will have a profound effect on your ability to adapt to change and your mental health.

Once Cassandra reappeared at the fairies' enchanted cottage, she observed them enjoying snacks and soft beverages while awaiting the completion of baking the pies. How they made her think of herself. She immediately directed them to clear up and dispose of any leftover snacks and processed foods. She told them to consume healthily and assisted them in creating a diet plan. Included were an exercise regimen and the objective of losing weight so that they could once again fly like fairies do. Cassandra would visit them periodically to keep them accountable and on track.

CHAPTER EIGHTEEN:
Final Words

Neuron Therapy and Metaphysical and Quantum Therapy (MQT) are the techniques I devised to make it simpler for my clients to connect with their neurons and make the necessary inner changes. Numerous clients and my coworkers use these terms to describe the work I perform. These methods have become commonplace in my social circle when discussing accessing the inner world.

Neuron Therapy (NT) is a type of psychotherapy that employs visualization and guided imagery techniques to transform or modify faulty thought patterns and behaviours from the inside by making direct contact with neurons. Neuron therapy is conducted in the presence of the therapist.

Metaphysical and Quantum Therapy (MQT) is a method of consciously and visually investigating your neurons, resulting in inner changes. This is an extension of neuron therapy that is quite similar to it, but also emphasizes the spiritual and mystical aspects of life. This method does not require the presence of the therapist. MQT can be completed independently. Those who adhere to esoteric or related teachings appear to embrace MQT and report significant changes from a non-scientific perspective. Later, if all goes as planned, we marry, if you will, the spiritual and material realms to bring about a long-overdue change.

You should now have a basic understanding of brain neurons, and I hope I have enlightened you on an alternative method to approach your mental health. As stated previously, not everyone will respond to the methods presented in this book, but the same is true of many other aspects of life. Not everyone responds to theories and practises supported by empirical evidence, and not everyone finds psychotherapy beneficial. Everyone is unique and responds differently to the various available strategies. Therefore, my recommendation is to discover something that works and stick with it.

I will now briefly conclude the accounts of those courageous clients who granted permission for their accounts to be shared. All the people mentioned in this book have successfully dealt with their mental health issues or are at least leading a richer life than before. To live contented and fruitful lives, ongoing maintenance and attention are required because we are all works in progress. Neuron Therapy is typically used in conjunction with other treatments or as a last resort when other treatments have failed. Always keep in mind that things do not always operate in a predictable or mechanical manner based on evidence. Occasionally, we must embrace the unknown and place our faith there as well. The evidence of this enigmatic aspect of our humanity is intensifying. Where attention goes, energy flows. And energy can be either healing or destructive, depending on your intentions. So be careful what you wish for!

If you recall, Cynthia's strategy was to use the ship as a vessel on the ocean to contact her neural world. She reported that she was flying high above the ship and that her inner world consisted of billions of neurons that resembled Shanghai at night. Remember that to free herself from her physical constraints and encounter her elusive Other Self, she had to stare nothingness in the face. She compared her damaged neurons to infants needing their mother to nurse them back to health, and this analogy proved effective for Cynthia. In her imagination, she was the mother bringing back to life her children (damaged neurons). The rational and neutral messages she was sending to her broken neurons were new codes, superseding the old, faulty, and damaging codes and messages that caused her anxiety and negative outcomes. Thus, by providing care and comfort to her defective neurons, she was, on a deeper 'unconscious' level, providing care and comfort to herself. Also, by safeguarding her vulnerable neurons, she safeguarded her vulnerable self. By repairing and strengthening her intelligent brain cells, Cynthia became more resilient. And by instructing Cynthia's neurons to maintain a healthy firing symphony, they had to arm themselves with psychological tools so they could defend themselves from being hacked. By learning these new strategies, Cynthia was also protecting and shielding herself in the outer world as well. Neuron Therapy was introduced to Cynthia because other forms of therapy did not work for her. Skills training did work well for her, but neuron therapy brought everything together for Cynthia.

Let us summarize the sessions of young Ben. Ben, age nine, contacted his neurons using soccer players, and then externalized them using illustrations on paper. He drew portraits and assigned them names such as Mr. Angry and Mr. Stupid and so forth. He also coloured his illustrations to convey their emotions. For example, his favourite colours would represent powerful and renowned soccer players, while his least favourite colours would represent neurons that were weak and afraid. His mission was to help those stupid neurons to become clever, and the frightened neurons to become brave. We also worked in twos, that is, having two similar neurons, as this made it easier for Ben to manage. If he was unable to change one of them, he would change the other one using a different method, and he would experience a sense of accomplishment regardless of the outcome of the first attempt. The effort was the reward. Focusing on and attempting to alter his thought processes and behaviour was the prize. Sometimes the journey is more important than the destination.

Ben was introduced to Neuron Therapy because other forms of therapy were ineffective for him. Ben benefited from training in basic and practical skills, but he eventually reverted to his negative thought patterns and self-defeating behaviours. Ben benefited from Neuron Therapy because it stimulated his creativity and maintained his interest in the sessions. He wanted to assist those neurons improve their soccer skills. He once told me that he compared his neural world to a large stadium filled with thousands of spectators witnessing an incredible soccer match, and that he was one of the greatest soccer players of all time.

Regarding the case of young Ben, the therapeutic alliance between the therapist and client was evident. Ben's psychological well-being and growth were significantly influenced by the therapeutic relationship between me and Ben.

Ben may require ongoing support in the future, but at the time of writing this book, he has undergone significant mental health improvements. His parents and teachers are amazed by his transformation, and they now describe him as a cheerful and delightful boy.

Stephen also made substantial progress, and if you recall, teenage Stephen used the cabin in the woods to connect with his neurons. He sat in front of a peculiar mirror and constructed a virtual world within it. Interestingly, he also subconsciously imagined those individuals hiding in the bushes and seemingly searching for something. Where did these inventions originate? At the time, it was a mystery to both of us. Were they attempting to warn Stephen about a growth occurring in his head? If we can access these communications, do our brains contain a built-in warning device system that alerts us of something?

Stephen has become hooked on the science of psychology and has turned his life around. Stephen is a pleasant and intelligent young man, and his mother keeps asking me what I did with her son. The young man that looks like Stephen is not her son because of his new positive and mature attitude and personality. What happened to that aggressive, anxious, and unhappy sixteen-year-old? Interestingly, though, Stephen related his inner world to resembling the universe, with billions of stars twinkling in the distance. When he brought his neural world to life in the mirror, he reported feeling as if he were in space, observing an infinite and unending universe.

Stephen was introduced to Neuron Therapy because other forms of therapy had failed to help him. Neuron Therapy was effective for him because it tapped into a deeper layer of his being. Stephen grew tired of conventional methods and desired a fresh approach to sink his teeth into. Neuron Therapy was new and fascinating to him, maintaining his interest. Additionally, he desired to conquer the neurons in his mirror. He wanted victory to transform them. Flying through space at the speed of light was too enticing for him. Significant and favourable changes can also be reported here. Stephen is on the right path, and his future looks promising.

The Black Dog is a common metaphor for someone suffering from severe depression. Patrick was one such person. He had almost given up on life because nothing worked for him. He was despondent. Over the years, he had attempted psychotherapy, medication, and alcohol, and not necessarily in that order. Numerous physicians, psychiatrists, psychologists, nutritionists, and naturopaths had been consulted. He altered his diet and way of life, embraced yoga, participated in meditation classes, and followed numerous recommendations made by concerned professionals and family members. At one point, he was also a vegetarian. But to no avail. His disposition remained depressed, and he cut himself off from his family and friends.

Patrick was introduced to Neuron Therapy because we believed he had nothing to lose. I found it difficult to encourage him to attend therapy and counselling. His wife was on my side, and we both held him accountable when I observed him having difficulty maintaining his appointments with me.

If you recall, we used diving as the 'entry' point into his neural universe. Those orange-spotted fish represented his neurons, while the deep-sea beast represented his black dog. I observed how he covertly attempted to protect his damaged neurons, which were his fish. He extracted them from the lake and placed them in a pool of water between the boulders at the water's edge. He intended to save them from the jaws of the sea monster.

Patrick has made an extraordinary recovery, and his wife cannot believe the transformation. Surprisingly, Patrick has resumed diving. He has become so motivated that he discussed teaching scuba diving to students. In his youth, Patrick was an avid diver who was constantly in the water. According to his wife, he has a new lease on life. The enormous fish tank he recently purchased was not what she wanted for the home, but she conceded because she had her husband back.

Patrick continues to communicate with me; in fact, many of my clients do so via email and snail mail, updating me on their progress and major life events. I also recall the day Patrick compared his neural world to the heavenly kingdom. Although Patrick was raised Catholic and attended Catholic schools as a child, he rarely discussed religion. As a result, I found this remark surprising. He explained that when he was underwater and surrounded by thousands of small fish, it was as if he entered a deeper state of mind, a tranquility he had never experienced before. He stated that it was as if the physical world had simply vanished. It felt surreal, as if time had abruptly halted; 'Like I was floating in pure silence, with everything hushed, and different hues of soft light all about, as if protecting and nourishing me, all in total, freaky silence, except that there was nothing freaky about this scene; it was simply blissful and loving.' The experience was so incredible that it moved Patrick to tears.

Jacquie is a well-groomed, professional woman in her late thirties who will shortly turn forty years old. She was losing hope of ever finding love and having a family. She disclosed that she was resigning herself to being single and alone for the remainder of her existence. She added that she would share her life with a few houseplants and some type of animal. She had no suitors, and that was that.

Remember that I suggested she use symbolism to enter her neural world because she struggled with visualization and self-hypnosis. She told me that she has a wandering mind. Therefore, we decided on the cluster of grapes, something creative that would allow her to utilize her drawing skills. I suggested that she draw a bunch of grapes dangling from a vine and give each grape a name. Individual grapes represented her neurons, while the grape vine represented her neural networks and interior world.

The broken grapes with sad expressions were Jacquie's clients as she joyfully assumed the therapist's role. She intended to help them through counselling. First, she had to determine the cause of their sadness. Then, she had to rewrite a new message to replace the unhelpful one that was written on the sorrowful grape. Inadvertently at first, Jacquie was identifying more erroneous messages as she worked through her grapes, and she eventually realized that she had to modify numerous messages to repair the grapes, which were, of course, her neurons.

During Jacquie's consultations, I witnessed numerous revelations as she pieced together how her damaged neurons were affecting her life. I could see her face light up as she replaced their negative codes, her flawed thought patterns, with something more beneficial and self-calming. I also observed her shedding tears when she thought I wasn't looking as she recalled yet another memory of some type. And it was at this point that I realized neuron therapy was the best course of action, as Jacquie was finally making progress. She told me that she had never delved so deeply into her psyche before and was feeling a sense of accomplishment. Challenging, but with a sense of achievement. She explained that it was as if she had been reborn.

This woman has undergone several transformations. She still has some distance to travel, but she is on the correct path. Jacquie reported feeling more at ease with herself and having resolved numerous psychological issues from her past. She also stated that she is a complicated woman who is nevertheless a marvellous work in progress. I like that comment.

I prompted Jacquie to summarize her thoughts at the conclusion of her therapy because she did not explain how she interpreted her inner world and working with neurons using symbolism. She eventually told me that her blank canvas represented her brain, and the paintings, drawings, sketches, and inscriptions on it represented her neurons. This large bunch of black grapes was the key that allowed her to enter her mind. In other words, the grapes served as an association to alert her that she would be entering her inner world to interact with her neurons.

Matthew had exhausted all options for managing his condition. Many older individuals will associate post-traumatic stress disorder (PTSD) with shell shock. If you recall, he lost a school companion when he was sixteen years old while on a school trip. Later, in his twenties, he was the victim of a robbery and gun attack. His life took a turn for the worse, and he ended up living alone in an apartment that his parents had purchased for him. He ultimately turned to drugs and alcohol as coping mechanisms to avoid reliving these traumatic events.

Matthew was introduced to Neuron Therapy because, frankly, nothing else was helping him, and he was on the fast track to mental collapse and, as he describes it, the cemetery.

We used his childhood home as a point of entry into his mind, as he recalled fond memories of growing up there. He adored all ball-based sports, so we utilized balls to contact his neurons. He lived on the foreshore of Sydney Harbour, he resided in a mansion that was surrounded by other enormous houses. At the end of the garden, the residence had its own private sandy beach. In addition, they had a boathouse with direct access to the water.

Matthew used his fond childhood recollections to overcome the fearful neurons he had developed because of past traumas. He required strength and courage to confront these fear-generating neurons. These neurons repeatedly replayed memories and images of his best friend's drowning and his assault at the liquor store. Other meaningless events since then that involved some drama were enlarged and twisted into something catastrophic, complete overreactions, thereby feeding, and securing his belief that the world was an unsafe and unenjoyable place; that something terrible was awaiting to end of him.

The balls represented his neurons, and he had to rinse and sanitize some of them because they were significantly soiled and worn. Some required air. Matthew was responsible for cleaning and reshaping the balls. Each ball was connected to a specific traumatic memory. The balls were recoded, reworded, and modified by cleaning and infusing them with positive and inspiring information. Eventually, these neurons would no longer transmit these traumatic messages and would instead transmit new, neutral messages, no longer causing him anxiety or continuously activating his fight-or-flight response system.

Interestingly, he compared his neural universe to that of his youth. He had difficulty explaining what he meant, but it was clear that as a child he felt secure and free and had an optimistic outlook on life. As the idiom goes, he was perpetually energized and content; the world was his oyster. Additionally, he felt invincible, always protected, and prosperous. He reported that his childhood was not only enchanted, but also the most wonderful period of his life.

Matthew's eyes would light up whenever he spoke of Isabella; she was a delightful addition. The woman was hesitant for me to include any information about her in this book, so only pertinent information about her is included. For the time being, I will only say that Matthew is in a relationship. Matthew is performing remarkably well, and he continues to keep me informed. Finally, his childhood residence is still standing with only minor modifications.

Cassandra used her bath to enter her neuron world and compared her neurons and neural networks to an enchanted forest where fairies lived. When interacting with their quantum world, each individual will encounter unique landscapes and describe unique scenarios. In Cassandra's case, the objective was to heal herself from the inside, from a quantum (microscopic or inner) perspective, which would increase her vibrational frequency to its proper level. Furthermore, whatever works for the client will be effective. Cassandra characterized her neural kingdom as resembling childhood fairy tales and, in later years, online computer games, giving her the impression that she was living in a supernatural forest or a computer game.

It was also intriguing how the two fat fairies mirrored Cassandra's existence. This realization unnerved Cassandra, and I believe it was one of the deciding factors in her decision to make life adjustments.

Cassandra was introduced to Neuron Therapy because other approaches and plans were not working. She repeatedly relapsed and was becoming disillusioned with support services and the possibility of change. Cassandra is an intelligent woman who, unfortunately, has used her intelligence to undermine every aspect of her world. She was oblivious that she consistently set herself up for failure. Her only solace in her miserable existence was food.

Cassandra gained the motivation to make modifications after overcoming her troublesome neurons and assuming the role of queen in her make-believe kingdom. Cassandra wished to help the two chubby fairies by giving them special consideration. So, she not only invited herself to their humble abode, but also ended up entering the neurons and erasing the self-defeating messages emblazoned on their inner walls. Finally, Cassandra described her neural world as resembling a fantasy land populated by whimsical, nonjudgmental, and harmless magical beings.

All the individuals mentioned in this book have, at some point, undergone mainstream and evidence-based therapies. All the clients discussed in this book have also attempted various forms of psychotherapy and other forms of support, including medication. Neuron Therapy was only used as a last resort, and typically only when other approaches or treatments had failed.

At the time of composing this book, the individuals mentioned are living happy, fruitful lives. All their prognoses are positive. They have embraced neuron therapy and thoroughly enjoyed working on themselves from the inside out.

Good luck and thank you for reading this book!

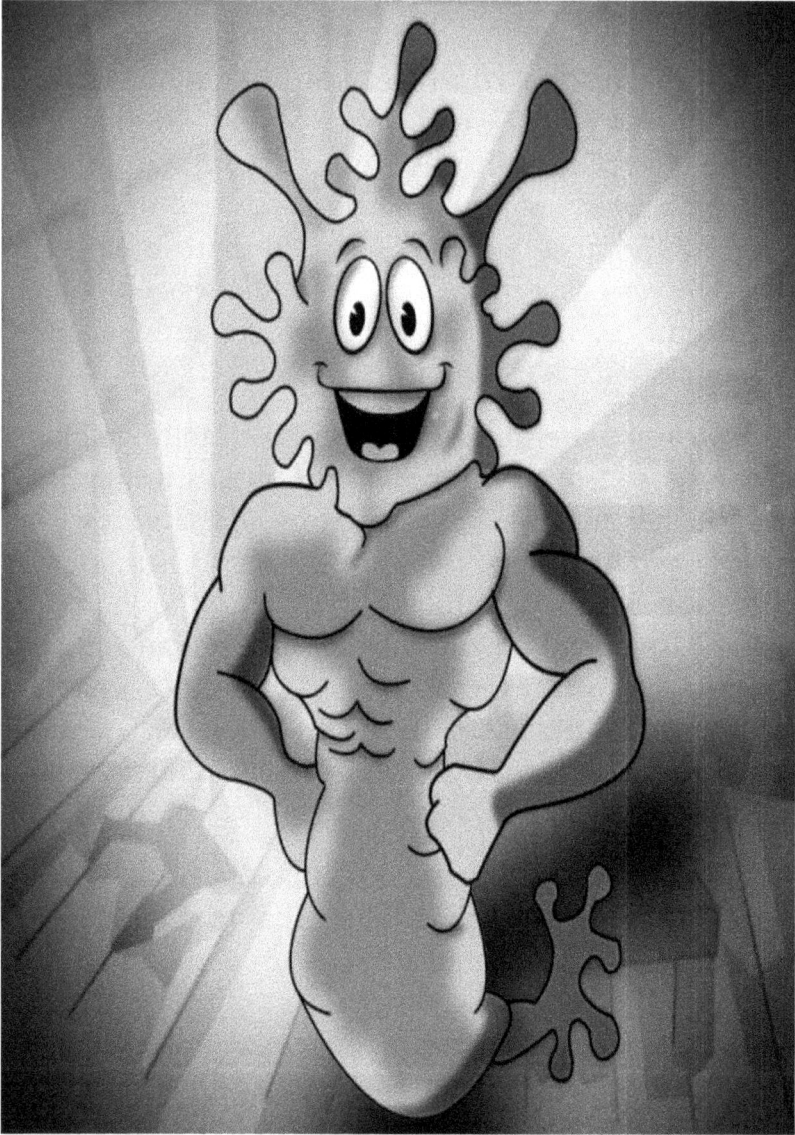

About the Author

Anthony is a sought-after and dynamic psychologist. He has over 25 years of experience and has always worked in the field of mental health. His clients describe him as popular, likeable, and intelligent, always striving to find solutions to their sometimes difficult and complex psychological issues. He believes that humour is the first step to getting back on track. In addition, Anthony is competent in all forms of anxiety management for children, adolescents, and adults.

Anthony has served as a consultant on many projects over the years and supervises numerous professionals in the mental health field. His training programs range from assertiveness training and personal development to identity rescue. He has developed new strategies for managing challenging behaviour when evidence-based practises and other conventional solutions fail. He is also innovative in his approach and constantly seeks the best results for his clientele.

In conclusion, Anthony Engel has always been interested in the mental health of people, young and old, and he continues to follow the most recent developments in psychology, such as Neuroscience and Neuroplasticity. Neuron Therapy is just one of his many creations.

The author can be contacted at analyst2@bigpond.com

www.ingramcontent.com/pod-product-compliance
Lightning Source LLC
Chambersburg PA
CBHW072134020426
42334CB00018B/1798

* 9 7 8 0 6 4 6 8 3 2 0 3 6 *